Praise for *Karate Science*

"Dr. Swanson makes a valuable contribution in understanding the how and why behind Shotokan karate techniques and principles. This book will help every martial artist better understand how the body works during martial movements, and how to generate strong, fast, and efficient techniques. *Karate Science: Dynamic Movement* is a great addition to any martial art library, and a must-read for those who practice Shotokan karate."

> —Alain Burrese, J.D.; fifth dan, Hapkido; author, *Hard-Won Wisdom from the School of Hard Knocks, Lost Conscience*; DVDS: *Hapkido Hoshinsul, Hapkido Cane, Streetfighting Essentials*

"Well, as you might expect from an associate professor of biology and biomedical sciences, this book is heavy on detail; however, because it is so well written, it is clear and concise, so you don't need to be a professor to read it. I found myself nodding in agreement on many occasions as I worked my way through the chapters, in particular [those regarding] the biomechanics involved in the practice and application of karate techniques. Obviously an accomplished karateka and instructor, Dr. Swanson has managed to produce a very comprehensive and useful resource to any student or instructor, and I would recommend its addition to any serious martial artist's library."

> —Aidan Trimble, eighth dan; chairman and chief instructor to the Federation of Shotokan Karate; former world karate champion (Tokyo 1983); author, *The Advanced Karate Manual*; *Karate Kata and Applications, Volumes 1, 2, 3, and 4*; *Karate for Kids*; *Fundamental Karate*; DVDs: *Applied Karate Series, Volumes 1, 2, and 3*

"Professor Swanson's book, *Karate Science: Dynamic Movement*, is written in such a way that it's easy to comprehend and applicable to all levels of karate practitioner. Instructors and students alike would benefit from reading this book and incorporating its clearly explained principles into their teachings and training. I am excited to use *Karate Science: Dynamic Movement* as the textbook for the karate course I teach at Temple University, Philadelphia."

> —Hiroyoshi Okazaki, eighth dan; author; chairman and chief instructor of the International Shotokan Karate Federation

"This is a *great* book! . . . This book cuts through the many misunderstandings and myths that surround Shotokan and gives technical, scientific, undisputable, and easily understood information for karateka of any level. It will allow readers to take this knowledge of the core principles and get back into the dojo to get on with the physical training that will help convert academic knowledge into physical intelligence. It is just what the Western karateka has been looking for."

—Scott Langley, sixth dan; chief instructor of World
Traditional Karate Organisation, Great Britain and
Ireland; author of *Karate Stupid* and *Karate Clever*

"This well-informed book demonstrates and explains how to apply the relevance and principles of biomechanics to a selected physical activity: karate. . . . I highly recommend all levels of karateka obtain this publication, as it will help all of us invaluably with our technique and teaching ability. This is a great read, and I've learned great things from it."

—Mark Willis, recipient, New Zealand Order of Merit;
seventh dan; deputy chief instructor, Traditional Shotokan
Karate-Do Federation; New Zealand country representative,
International Shotokan Karate Federation

"I had the pleasure of meeting Dr. J. D. Swanson when he first came to the United States of America in 1998. It was clear from my first meeting with him that he is an intelligent individual who is passionate about all aspects of his life, whether it is his academics, family, or karate. It is that same combination of intelligence and passion that Dr. Swanson brings to *Karate Science: Dynamic Movement.* If you're interested in the sizzle and not the steak, may I suggest you go someplace else. However, if you are looking for practical and scientifically insightful guidance about Shotokan karate and the superior executions of its movements, this is a must-read."

—Carl Shaw, M.Ed, MBE; eighth dan, ISKF

"*Karate Science: Dynamic Movement* is an outstanding, complete, and detailed work. The author covers a range of fundamental principles and technical subtleties that are critical to learning, understanding, and applying karate's physical principles. This book has something to offer beginner through advanced practitioners, as well as instructors looking for new ways to develop and coach their students."

—Edmond Otis, eighth dan; chairman and chief instructor,
AJKA-International; author, *Complete Idiot's Guide to
Karate*, with Randall Hassell; DVDs: *Essential Shotokan*
video series

"The book is a concise and valuable source of reference for those wishing to further their study of karate. Techniques are described not only in terms of the underlying biomechanical principles, but explained from the performer's

internal perspective. Theoretical explanations are no substitute for 'discovery through training,' but this ambitious work is a welcome addition, which serious martial artists should be happy to add to their bookshelves."
—David Hooper, PhD; associate editor, *Classical Fighting Arts*

"J. D. has written an entertaining and insightful book looking at karate from the perspective of a scientist and has succeeded in the difficult task of making the science approachable. The book has a refreshing take, as it addresses karate technique in a questioning manner that encourages thought and contemplation in the reader. By focusing on conveying the feeling of 'how to' technique rather than just the shape of technique, deeper thought and analysis are possible, which have been presented here with excellent imagery, analogies, and some stimulating mind maps. If you read this book, you should not only gain a greater understanding of some of the dynamics of karate, but you should gain a greater understanding of how you can further your own analysis and thus development of karate."
—Dr. Matthew Pain, reader in biomechanics, School of Sport, Exercise and Health Sciences, Loughborough University, United Kingdom

"I have always loved the energy and enthusiasm that Dr. Swanson exhibits in everything he does, including karate. Therefore, I am pleased to see this very technical and educational publication come to fruition. I especially enjoyed the sections explaining the forces that come into play during stance training and shifting. The illustrations were also helpful in visualizing how the hips 'react' during expansion and contraction. I assisted Okazaki Shihan and Dr. Stricevic in editing their *Textbook of Modern Karate* back in the eighties, and this book provides some different images and ideas that I find refreshing and helpful. I know I have come away with new teaching ideas after reading *Karate Science: Dynamic Movement.*"
—Cathy Cline, eighth dan; regional director, ISKF Northwest Region; chief instructor, Western Washington Shotokan Karate Club; secretary, ISKF Technical Committee

"Swanson's debut is a scientific guide to the stances, movements, and techniques of karate.

"Swanson, a professor of biology and biomechanics at Salve Regina University, uses his scientific training to help teachers and students better understand the tenets of karate. The many illustrations (ably provided by Nigro) show everything from proper alignment of a striking surface (say, a fist or a foot) to how one's body should move from the beginning to the end of a thrust.

The first part of the book focuses on technique, with sections on stances, thrusting, kicking, striking, and blocking. The guide does more than demonstrate how positions should look; Swanson takes the time to explain how each should feel and which muscle groups should be engaged throughout the process. The second part explains the science behind how our joints and muscles work, as well as how the body keeps its balance. This section also includes a brief primer on 'the application of kinesiological principles to karate,' which outlines ways to get more force into moves by increasing mass, and, crucially, speed. The last section deals with the notion of 'internal movement,' essentially a system of muscle retraction and countermoves that aid in perfecting efficient and powerful techniques. While many students mistakenly think of this process as simply hip wiggling, Swanson shows that the process is more focused on intra-abdominal pressure, and he explains how the proper tensioning and contracting of certain muscles are key to quick and powerful movements. Swanson's writing is clear and informative, and his pure love of the art shines through. This book is not for karate neophytes, and the terms used will be confusing to unfamiliar readers. But for teachers and students who want to not only perfect techniques, but also understand the biology behind them, the book will be an invaluable aid.

"An informative guide for those looking to enhance their karate training."
—*Kirkus Reviews*

KARATE SCIENCE

DYNAMIC MOVEMENT

J. D. SWANSON, PHD

YMAA Publication Center
Wolfeboro, NH USA

YMAA Publication Center, Inc.
PO Box 480
Wolfeboro, New Hampshire 03894
1-800-669-8892 • info@ymaa.com • www.ymaa.com
ISBN: 9781594394591 (print) • ISBN: 9781594394607 (ebook)

Edited by Doran Hunter
Cover design by Axie Breen
Illustrated by Sam Nigro
This book is typeset in Adobe Garamond and Frutiger

0118

Publisher's Cataloging in Publication

Name: Swanson, J. D. (John-David), 1973- author.
Title: Karate science : dynamic movement / J. D. Swanson. —
Description: Wolfeboro, NH USA : YMAA Publication Center, [2017] | Includes bibliographical
    references and index.
Identifiers: ISBN: 9781594394591 (print) | 9781594394607 (ebook) | LCCN: 2016962683
Subjects: LCSH: Karate—Training. | Karate—Physiological aspects. | Human mechanics. | Biomechanics. |
    Martial arts—Training. | Martial arts—Physiological aspects. | Hand-to-hand fighting, Oriental—
    Training. | Hand-to-hand fighting, Oriental-Physiological aspects. | BISAC: SPORTS &
    RECREATION / Martial Arts & Self-Defense. | SCIENCE / Applied Sciences. | SPORTS &
    RECREATION / Training.
Classification: LCC: GV1114.33.T72 S93 2017 | DDC: 796.815/3—dc23

Printed in USA.

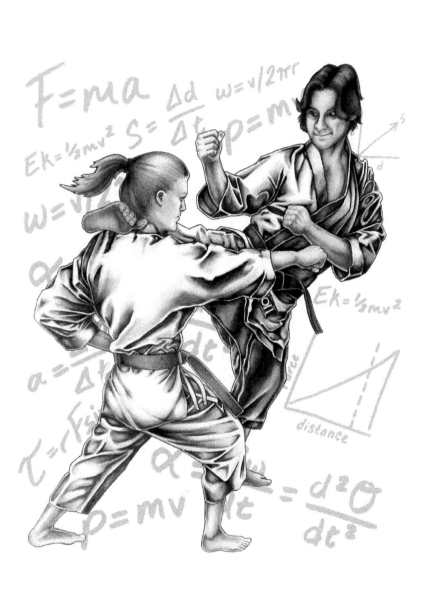

EDITORIAL NOTES

The spelling and pronunciation of certain transliterated Japanese terms vary by context. *Tsuki*, for example, is a class of hand techniques. When this term appears with a modifier describing the technique, tsuki becomes *zuki*. *Oi zuki*, therefore, is a lunge punch.

Keri is the Japanese term for kick. When used with a modifier, keri becomes *geri*, which is why a front kick is *mae geri*. The word *geri* alone means diarrhea.

TABLE OF CONTENTS

PART III

Internal Movement of Karate   163

FOREWORD

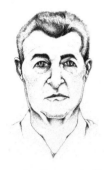

Robin Rielly, eighth dan, International Shotokan Karate Federation

It gives me great pleasure to see this book in print. In today's market there is no shortage of books on karate, many by well-known experts in the field. This work is different. For the first time we have the observations of a karate instructor who is skilled in both the scientific field of biology as well as in karate. Professor J. D. Swanson is a longtime practitioner of karate and a certified instructor, judge, and examiner for the International Shotokan Karate Federation. He brings to the discussion a wealth of information that will help the karateka understand how and why the body moves in certain ways during the performance of stances, punches, strikes, blocks, and kicks. The book offers fresh insights into how the various muscle groups interact during the execution of these movements. In addition, the reader will be made aware of various methods of training the body that will improve karate techniques from both mental and physical approaches.

This work will be a significant resource for both instructors and their students. Instructors will have the scientific rationale available for the teaching of karate movements and how their students must perform them. Students will have an additional source of information to supplement their regular instructor's lessons.

Many instructors are proficient in teaching movements to their students. However, for a good number, their proficiency is based on constant repetition, rather than a thorough understanding of how the body actually works. Professor Swanson's approach fills a much-needed gap for instructors and students alike. In order to utilize one's body efficiently, it is necessary to understand the factors that generate strong, fast, and correct movement. Throughout the book, Professor Swanson gives valuable suggestions to help maximize body efficiency.

In all, I believe that this is one of the most important books on the practice of karate that has been published in recent years. The International Shotokan Karate Federation has continued to grow and prosper through the efforts of both the older generation of instructors and the younger ones who continually strive to improve our knowledge as we continue to develop and grow into the twenty-first century. Thanks to the work of instructors such as Professor Swanson, we will continue to make progress in our study of karate.

ROBIN L. RIELLY
Eighth dan, ISKF
Member, Shihankai (ISKF)
Chairman, ECSKA Technical Committee

FOREWORD

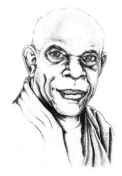

James Field, eighth dan, International Shotokan Karate Federation

In karate a straight punch is executed with snap efficiency and shoots straight to the target. This book by J. D. Swanson does the same. Chapters are short, efficient, and to the point. They have solid content and make an impact.

Dr. Swanson approaches the subject of karate from a unique personal perspective that is both thoughtful and thought provoking. Here's a sample description of kiba dachi (or horse-riding) stance: "The feeling is as if the practitioner is pushing on a flexible bow braced down the inside of the leg and attached to the hip and foot. As the practitioner pushes down, the bow bows outward, creating the bend in the knee. Kiba dachi is formed by two of these bows pushing toward each other, hence the stability of the stance." Now, that's a simple description that's clear and easy to picture, yet I've never heard it before in my fifty-plus years of practicing Shotokan karate. I believe it's a really helpful explanation.

Whenever possible, Dr. Swanson attempts to explain the *why* behind karate body positions and body dynamics (important and often neglected information in karate books). For example, he doesn't just say to keep the back leg straight but not locked in a forward stance, but adds why: if the rear leg is locked, "this will lift the rear hip and break the lower back posture by lifting the buttock up and out." Or, "if the technique requires a bend in the elbow, then a ninety-degree angle is best" because "the right angle presents the strongest position for the biceps to keep the arm bent due to utilizing the maximum number of filaments interacting in the muscle." The rules of biomechanics and physics as they apply to karate are frequently employed here.

From the description of how to make a fist to the discussion of how to reconcile the "seemingly paradoxical $F = ma$ equation used in karate," there is something here to be learned for practitioners at every level.

This book is well researched, well illustrated, and should prove an excellent tool in promoting the understanding of the art of karate.

I am happy to recommend it.

JAMES FIELD
Eighth dan, ISKF
Member, Shihankai (ISKF)
Director, ISKF Technical Committee
Director and chief instructor, ISKF Southwest Region

ACKNOWLEDGMENTS

J. D. SWANSON

I would first like to thank everyone involved in the writing of this manuscript. That includes Pat, Rick, Maddie, and Arison for the first proofs. Sensei Robin Rielly offered careful and insightful comments in later drafts, and Sensei Steve Ubl provided the finishing touches. I was so much more nervous about giving this manuscript to the two of you than I was my PhD thesis to my advisors.

Now for making this book what it really is, thanks to Sam Nigro. What started as a harebrained idea—"I want some pics that show the X, Y, and Z of karate"—and you came up with this . . . Wow, just wow. Maddie and Michelle, thanks for posing with me for some of the pictures.

Thank you to the folks at YMAA, in particular Doran for his editing, T.G. for keeping me calm, and Barbara for keeping me on point. You all are awesome!

I would like to thank all of my instructors. Some of you I have known and trained with for many years, some for short periods, but all of you have helped me develop both in technique and understanding, inspiring me by walking the path ahead. In particular, some of you have truly taken me under your wing and dragged me back to the path. Thank you to Sensei Okazaki, Rielly, Ubl, Sill, Glucina, Vance, Pain, and Kalmancsi. Also, I would like to thank all of you who train with me day to day. I still can't believe you put up with me. I have seen you grow and develop in ways I never expected. All of you have had a profound impact on my life, and I am forever grateful.

Finally, I would like to thank my wife for understanding and supporting my karate obsession all these years. Thanks to my parents for driving me to class every day when I was young and providing the encouragement I needed, even when I wanted to give up. This would not exist with out you. Last but not least, thanks to my little "Mr. Human." This initial manuscript was written in a rush before you came into my life and will be published just a few weeks before your third birthday—and it is to you that I dedicate this first work.

SAM NIGRO

I would like to thank Dr. J. D. Swanson for offering me the opportunity to illustrate his new work. I would also like to thank him, Gerry Perrino, and Susannah Strong for their encouragement throughout my academic and artistic success.

Finally, I would like to thank both of my parents for their unconditional love and support throughout all of my endeavors.

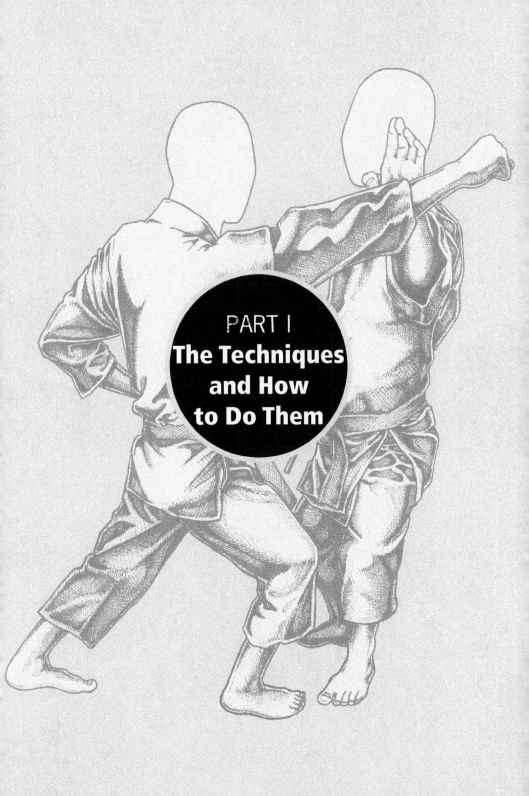

PART I
**The Techniques
and How
to Do Them**

CHAPTER 1

An Introduction and How to Use This Book

Introduction

The Asian martial arts have a rich history and present a variety of techniques and methods that can be used to incapacitate an opponent. The techniques used in the unarmed martial arts of Asia are of a much greater variety than many of the Western methods. Okazaki Sensei, one of my instructors and one of the world's most senior Shotokan karate instructors, tells the story of when he first came to the United States in the 1960s. It was arranged that he fight in a demonstration match in Philadelphia against a boxer. While the parties concerned were discussing the details of the fight, they were asked to demonstrate the types of techniques that would be used. The boxer gave a masterful demonstration of hooks, jabs, uppercuts, and crosses, while Okazaki Sensei demonstrated punching, striking, blocking, and kicking techniques from karate. The promoters immediately stepped in and requested that Okazaki limit his techniques to punches. Okazaki Sensei declined, stating that karate was the sum total of all of these techniques, and it would not be a true karate demonstration without them. The fight was canceled. While the outcome of the match could have gone either way, Okazaki's point was clear.

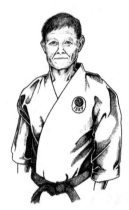

Okazaki Teruyuki, tenth dan, ISKF.

This book is about those techniques and, more importantly, my current interpretation of how to do them. While the techniques have been described many times, not much has been written about the technical detail behind the "how" of their performance or the way they "feel." In my own training, I have observed that much of this information is never taught, either on purpose or simply because the concepts were never taught to the instructor. This book attempts to rectify this. I will talk about the important parts of the body, how they need to be contracted or relaxed at the correct place and time, and the biomechanics involved. I have attempted to explain things in the same way I do in my own dojo, in a simple and clear manner. It is my hope that this will get you, the reader, thinking and looking deeper into your own martial arts training.

One important caveat is that the concepts discussed in this book represent my current way of thinking. Since I have been writing the first drafts of this book, I have learned more and more each day. My understanding and practice of karate, as for any serious student of the art, will inevitably evolve and change for the better. It is my sincere hope that readers of this book will learn, challenge themselves, and progress in their lifelong study of karate.

Differences between Asian and Western Training Methods

Many of my peers who have trained at length in Japan comment that training consists of simply doing thousands of repetitions in class with little or no instruction. The student does without question what the instructor commands. Judging from the ability level of these students, it is clear that this method works. However, it requires a complete acceptance of the Asian way of doing things. This way of training leads to an understanding of karate at the level of physical movements; that is, students may not know how a movement is done, but there is certainly no argument that they can do it.

Many of the early instructors from Japan found that Westerners did not take to that type of training. Many students quit after a short time. Okazaki Sensei relates that if he hadn't modified his training methods from what they were in Japan, his clubs would have dissolved. Unfortunately, language barriers made it hard for some of the Japanese instructors to communicate; therefore, explanations sometimes were not communicated well. This in turn led to some common technical mistakes that have been perpetuated in Western countries. These mistakes, which varied from organization to organization, could have arisen from several sources. The senior instructor could have overemphasized a particular concept, leading to the student thinking the exaggerated movement was the correct way to execute the technique. The instructors may simply have had flawed technique. Finally, they may have had a personal way of performing a technique that was correct for their body type that could have been passed to the student. A mistake can often be traced back to an original instructor, and even to a particular period of an instructor's teaching career.

Fortunately, Westerners have taken what they have learned from their Asian instructors and reflected very deeply and thoroughly on how karate is done. In addition, many of the native English-speaking karateka who have significant experience training in Japan have come back to their home countries and articulated what the first Japanese instructors could not. Also, there are many Westerners with a lifetime of experience. For all these reasons, there is now a wealth of sources for understanding karate. You can even make a strong case that in exploring karate unburdened by the baggage of cultural tradition, Western karateka have advanced karate from where it was in the 1960s. Arguably the best example of this is in kata application or bunkai. While many theories exist as to the proposed "initial intent" of kata bunkai, unrealistic applications were taught through the 1960s to 1980s. However, the application of kata has been revolutionized by the work of Schmeisser, Abernethy, Ubl, and others, which has led to a renaissance in our understanding of kata and how it can be applied in realistic situations.

With so much information available, it is very important not to confuse *cerebrally* understanding a karate technique with doing it. While long-term training in Japan involves a definite "it factor," this clearly comes from the rigorous, sustained training and immediate, abrupt feedback students receive. This method requires, however, a particular mindset and can take a very long time because there is no real direction as to what is correct. The student receives only visual guidance and nothing about the feeling or the *how* of the technique. On the other hand, if karateka spend a lot of time seeking explanations with not enough doing, they will not progress, because while the mind may understand, the body will not perform properly due to the lack of repetition. Therefore, it is my feeling that there must be a balance between understanding and physical training. And while the scale should always be tipped to the training side, a student should work to understand how a technique is done.

The analogy I like to use for this is basketball players practicing free throws. If they simply practice the physical act of throwing the ball into the basket, they may do well, but only after a time. Likewise, if they visualize in their mind the act and *feeling* of throwing the ball into the net, they will also succeed somewhat. But they will achieve the best and fastest results if their practice incorporates a combination of both actually throwing the ball and visualization. The cerebral part of the training allows the student not only to understand but also to jumpstart the process of internalizing the movement, which must then be drilled again and again until it is perfected.

How to Use This Book

As noted above, there is a lot of information on how karate techniques are performed. For example, consider the front stance, or zenkutsu dachi. The feet are shoulder width apart, with one foot one and a half to two shoulder widths in front of the other. Both feet face forward as much as the body's flexibility allows, with the front knee bent and the back leg straight. While this is an accurate description of how the stance should look, there is almost no information to be found about how it should feel, the dynamic tension held in this static

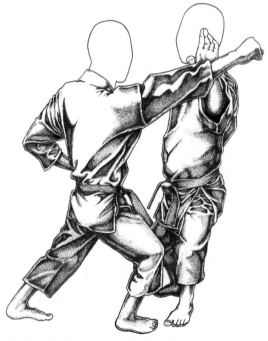

Blocking a lunge punch, or oi zuki, with a vertical knife-hand block, or tate shuto uke.

position. That dynamic tension allows the body weight to be used in the transition to the technique to be executed. Many people train in front of a mirror, but as many seasoned karateka know, the mirror is not required; it is simply a way to see the technique. A mirror can be detrimental to training if overused as it can put you outside yourself. Each technique has a particular *feeling*, and a change in the way a well-practiced technique feels can indicate that the technique is off. In some ways, I could describe this work as a book of feelings. These feelings and the biomechanical or anatomical principles they stem from are not often discussed in dojo, so I hope this book can provide further insight as you train. However, while I will describe these feelings and principles to you, it is up to you to experience them for yourself.

Throughout this book I have used anatomical terms for clarity. Some important ones are plantar flexing versus dorsiflexing of a limb. Simply put, plantar flexing is when the end of a limb is pointed flat out, in the direction of the limb, as when the toes are pointed. Plantar flexing is flat like a plane or flat surface. Dorsiflexing is when the end of the limb is bent perpendicular to the limb, as when the toes are pulled back toward the shinbone. Other common anatomical terms used here are supination and pronation. For example, if the arms are held by the side of the body and the thumb is stuck out like a hitchhiker, pronation is when the forearm is twisted in such a way that the thumb is pointing toward to the body, while supination is when the thumbs are pointing outward from the body.

This book has three major parts. The first part deals with the techniques themselves. In this section the primary techniques of karate are covered. Each is discussed in terms of both the final position (static) and the feeling that runs through the movements leading to the final position, as well as the feeling involved in the final position itself (dynamic). To do this I have used a standard way of organizing many of the techniques. Each class of technique—stances (dachi), thrusting or punching (tsuki), kicking (keri), striking (uchi), blocking (uke), and balance breaking (kuzushi)—has been broken down into separate chapters.

The second and third parts of the book focus on the core principles associated with generating power from all techniques. This includes several chapters on biomechanics and anatomy, kime, hip movement, and also different ways that we hit targets. In these chapters, some of the more nebulous or misunderstood concepts, such as "hip vibration" and kime, are discussed, defined, and explained in terms of how to do them in a clear manner.

While many examples originate from a Shotokan karate perspective, examples from other styles of karate including Goju-ryu, Wado-ryu, Uechi-ryu, as well as other martial arts such as aikido, taekwondo, and judo are also used. Many of the concepts in this book are applicable to any martial art. Simply put, there are only so many ways to move the human body; we are all governed by the same principles of dynamics.

Once again, it is my sincere hope that you read this book, agree with at least parts of it, learn something, argue with your friends, but, most importantly, use it as a springboard to make your training better and more efficient.

CHAPTER 2

The Four Fundamental Requirements of Martial Arts

Karate-do, or any other martial art, is, at its core quite simple. However, it can be made far more complex than what it actually is. The multitude of techniques, combinations, kata, and partner drills—combined with nebulous concepts like "use your hips," "lower your stance," "do budo karate," "make more kime," and "use your ki"—can make martial arts seem overwhelming. While the many concepts are important, they are often treated as doctrine in the teaching of karate. This can foster misconceptions and hamper understanding, and therefore practice, of karate, often for very long stretches of a student's training.

Additionally, when attending seminars, clinics, or even everyday class, students are often inundated by a multitude of techniques and spend much of their time simply trying to understand what is being taught. This may perhaps be the wrong approach. An example is the theming of individual lessons. It has become very popular to "theme" individual lessons: teach a single concept throughout. This could be a particular technique or group of techniques, such as tsuki or keri; individual concepts in training, such as polishing a kata or kata bunkai (application); or perhaps concepts or principles that relate to budo overall, such as the correct use of hips, timing, or posture. The latter is a far more advanced method of teaching karate and uses techniques (kihon), kata practice, and partner training (kumite) to illustrate and reinforce overall principles that show a practitioner *how* to do karate. If these principles are understood and followed, students will elevate their level overall.

So out of the multitude of principles available, which are the most important to learn? In conversations with some of my own high-ranking seniors, many agreed on certain points. But Sensei Steve Ubl (eighth dan, World Traditional Karate Organization) said it the most succinctly: in order to do karate effectively, there are four fundamental areas to be mastered: posture, structural alignment, body mechanics, and practical functionality.

Good Posture

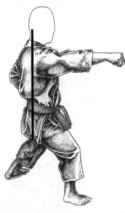

Perpendicular alignment of the back relative to the floor in oi zuki, or lunge punch.

Good posture is fundamental to all karate and martial arts practice. Posture refers to the back being straight from head to hips: The backbone is straight, the head sits atop the shoulders and is not slumped forward, the tailbone is tucked, and the pelvis is tilted in such a way that the lower back is straight. It is important not to have the lower back relaxed so that the buttocks stick out or are contracted too far so that the pelvis is pushed forward and under. Finally, note that having a straight back does not mean that it is perpendicular to the floor. It can be tilted relative to the floor, as long as it is straight from tailbone to head and it contributes to the structural integrity of the technique. A perfect example of this is in yama zuki, or mountain punch (see chapter 6).

Good Structural Alignment

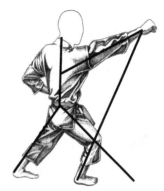

One of the main goals of karate is to have the body postured in such a way as to allow a direct connection from the floor to the striking limb at the point of impact. In fundamental karate this is how techniques such as oi zuki finish (see below). The final position, although held very briefly in a real encounter, is vitally important. These alignments provide the strongest position of the body for a particular technique or a particular target.

Structural alignment of oi zuki. Lines show direct connection from fist to floor.

Good Body Mechanics

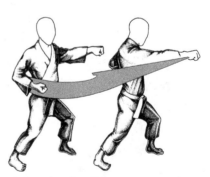

When we hear the term "oi zuki," or lunge punch, we often imagine a karate technique with one leg out in front and the arm on the same side out punching. However, if we only consider the final position of the technique as being the complete technique, we will have

Motion of gyaku zuki, or reverse punch, from preparatory position to final technique.

missed much of the point. The term oi zuki refers to the entire motion of a stepping punch from start to finish. In some ways the Japanese names of the techniques are verbs rather than nouns: they refer to motions and the body feeling of doing those motions.

However, being aware that the entire motion is important, *how* that motion is completed—especially with reference to its mechanics—is vital. Bruce Lee often talked about economy of motion. This concept simply means good body mechanics. By having good mechanics, martial artists will be faster, hit the target with much more force, and experience much less wear and tear on their bodies through training.

Good Practical Functionality

Good practical functionality refers to peripheral concepts such as distance, timing, and the resulting application of the technique. It is important to note that the three concepts outlined above (good posture, good structural alignment, and good body mechanics) all have to be adhered to first, then practical functionality can then be added.

Distancing, or maai, refers to the physical spatial relationship that two people share during an encounter. It changes constantly, and the length of limbs will alter what techniques may be thrown at any time. It is important for practitioners to consider both the length of their own maai (What can I hit them with right now?) and their partner's maai (What can I be hit with right now?) and learn how to control the distance to their advantage.

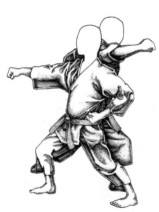

Evasion of a lunge punch, or oi zuki, by rotating around and finishing with an empi uchi, or elbow strike to the head.

Timing can refer to a multitude of things in karate. Initially, it can mean the mechanical requirements of a technique. For example, in a reverse punch, is the hand stopping as the hip stops moving, or have the hip and body center stopped moving, with the hand going on by itself? Obviously, it is best if the hip, body center, and hand all stop concurrently. Timing can also refer to the temporal relationship between opponents, that is, the timing involved in successfully launching or defending against an attack. Both timing and distance are intimately linked, and understanding the relationship between the two is paramount.

A well-founded knowledge of how each technique is applied is also vital for understanding karate, or any martial art. Once all of the above requirements are met, the technique may be practiced with a partner. This includes body positioning, foot positioning and entry, target acquisition, reaction of the target, and changing both practitioners' body positions after the application of the technique to set up for the next technique.

These four fundamental requirements need to be studied vigilantly in order to become proficient at karate, and martial arts in general. Each must be thoroughly mastered at an instinctual level. With this in mind, it could be said that the measure of your karate ability lies not necessarily in the number of techniques or kata you know, but rather in how good your fundamentals are. These fundamentals must become second nature, which can often only be achieved over a lifetime. One thing is certain: only through constant, vigilant practice can our body begin to understand these fundamentals.

CHAPTER 3

With What and How Do I Make a Hitting Surface?

The Asian martial arts are notable for the range of body parts used to strike an opponent. This range of weapons allows a greater variety of targets and angles practitioners can use to thrust (chapter 6), kick (chapter 7), strike (chapter 8), block (chapter 9), or generally make contact with an opponent. This chapter will review the major body parts used to strike an opponent.

While the parts used are important, and are the focus of this chapter, it is important to keep in mind that all body parts are used in karate. Of particular note are the hips, which are used as the fulcrum of body movement, as well as the abdominals, which connect the upper and lower body together. This will be discussed in depth in the second part of this book.

Ready-Made Weapons

Before we discuss the different weapons of the body, it is important to consider that some body parts are not ready-made for striking an opponent, and must be conditioned to do so. We may have to condition the weapon itself or its associated support structures to brace the weapon so it does not break upon impacting a target. A classic example is the fist. First the knuckles need to be conditioned to be able to take impact. Meanwhile, the wrist also needs to be conditioned so that it does not buckle. There are many ways to do this, but the most popular is to do pushups on the knuckles (seiken) that impact the target. This develops wrist strength and lets the bones in the hand receive stress in the distal and proximal direction,[1] providing a stimulus for the bones to remodel their internal architecture and withstand impact in that direction. Once this is achieved, it is important for the practitioner to hit targets. These must provide some feedback but not be so rigid as to cause damage. Makiwara or pad work can aptly serve this purpose.

Alternatively, there are some weapons, such as teisho (palm heel) or the heel or ball of the foot, that are already strong and can be used without conditioning. It is important to understand this difference quickly to lower the risk of injury when actually using the weapon.

Striking Points of the Hand and Wrist

The hand and wrist contain over seventeen different striking points. The sheer adaptability of the end of the limb makes it an incredibly versatile weapon that can be used at a variety of angles to strike a variety of targets.

---

1. "Distal" refers to the end of the limb that is far (distal) from the human body. "Proximal" refers to the end that is near it.

Seiken

The first weapon is seiken, or the forefist. This consists of the front knuckles of the index and middle fingers. In order to construct a correct fist, the fingers are rolled tightly, starting at the tips and progressively rolled downward into the fist. The fingers dig into the meaty part of the palm just above (not into) the first line in the hand, creating a strong compact ball. The thumb then pushes down firmly on the middle knuckle of the index and middle finger on the under-

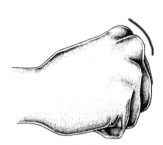

Seiken, or the forefist.

side of the fist. The strongest squeezing finger is the little finger, which should feel that it is winding both tighter and back toward the center of the hand.

The wrist must be held straight so that the knuckles of the hand leading from the index and middle finger are in line with the radius and ulna of the forearm. This can be observed when the hand is held straight and the fingers are flexed downward at the knuckle that connects the fingers to the hand to a right angle. The region of the hand between the wrist and knuckle naturally makes a slight upward angle that looks out of line to the forearm, but despite this angle, this is the correct alignment for the bones of the hand to connect to the

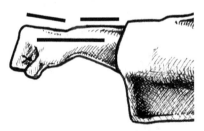

Correct wrist position of the fist.

forearm. This same angle must be maintained in the fist. Biomechanically, it is the strongest position for the hand and wrist when clenched in a fist. It is commonly taught that the top of the hand is in line with the top of the forearm (e.g., you could lay a ruler along the forearm and top of the fist), but this is incorrect and will lead to the wrist buckling downward and being injured if a target is hit. For openhanded techniques, if the hand is held flat, then the hand is held directly in line with the forearm.

As previously stated, seiken is not a ready-made weapon and needs conditioning of both the knuckles and wrist to allow it to be used effectively.

Uraken

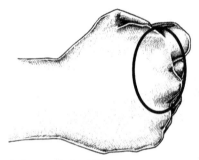

Uraken, or the backfist.

Uraken, or the backfist, is formed in the same way as seiken, but the back of the knuckles of the index and middle fingers are used. Generally, uraken is used when the radius and ulna are fully rotated to the supinated position. This is a fairly ready-formed weapon.

Tettsui

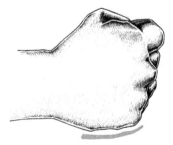

Tettsui, or the bottom fist.

Tettsui, or the bottom fist, is also formed the same way as seiken; however, the bottom of the fist is used (the surface provided by the curled little finger). This is a very strong ready-made weapon that can be used to strike hard surfaces.

Ippon-Ken

Ippon-ken, or the one-knuckle fist, is constructed the same way as seiken, but the index finger knuckle is extended out of the fist to make a point at the second finger joint. The thumb is moved to a higher position in the hand so that it presses onto the second joint, pushing both down in and away from the hand. It is a ready-made weapon for attacking precise soft vital points of the body.

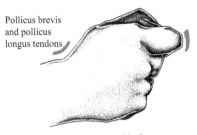

Pollicus brevis and pollicus longus tendons

Ippon-ken, or the one-knuckle fist.

This thumb position both provides support to the striking surface and stabilizes the wrist. This is through both the *pollicus brevis* and *pollicus longus* tendons that connect the thumb to the wrist. The tightening of these tendons through their associated muscles can greatly stabilize the wrist, and this is why many hand positions have the thumb in this position.

This alternative thumb position is used in the seiken position in other types of karate, such as in Isshin-ryu. This is because this style of karate was often taught to Marines visiting Okinawa, who did not have years to develop the correct muscles in the wrist. Using these two tendons was an easier and quicker method to develop wrist stabilization. In contrast, seiken used in Shotokan karate does not have the thumb in this position and really only makes use of the *pollicus brevis* to stabilize the wrist. However, through several years of training, the muscles of the forearm and underside of the wrist are developed, creating a much better stabilizing position. When compared to a fully strengthened and conditioned wrist, this alternative thumb position is not as stable.

Nakadate-Ippon-Ken

In nakadate-ippon-ken, or the middle finger one knuckle, the middle knuckle is extended to expose the point of the second joint of the middle finger. The thumb and little

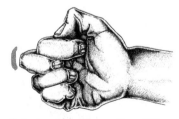

Nakadate-ippon-ken, or the middle finger one knuckle.

finger squeeze the weapon together in a fashion similar to seiken. It is a ready-made weapon for attacking precise soft vital points of the body.

Hiraken

Hiraken, or the fore-knuckle fist, has the same wrist setup as seiken; however, the entire hand is extended so that the striking surface is the points of the second knuckle joints of the hand. It is a ready-made weapon used to slot into narrow spaces, such as the *philtrum* or throat.

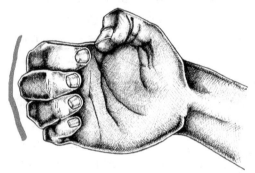

Hiraken, or the fore-knuckle fist.

There are two ways to create this weapon. The first is where the hand is flat to the second knuckle joint with the thumb bent. The second is the same position as ippon-ken. All knuckles are extended so that the fingers form a triangle when looking down at the thumb side of the hand. In this second configuration, the thumb is able to support by pushing in and out from the hand. Either position is satisfactory for wrist support, since the *pollicus brevis* and *pollicus longus* tendons are employed due to the position of the thumb. The weapon is braced by the flat alignment into the hand, the thumb pushing into the index finger.

Teisho

Teisho, or palm heel, is constructed the same way as the

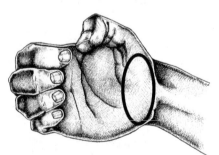

Teisho, or palm heel.

flat version of hiraken, but the wrist is extended upward, exposing the meaty part of the palm. This is a very strong ready-made weapon.

Kumade

Kumade, or bear hand, is constructed the same way as the flat version of hiraken. The weapon is the palm and can be used to attack the face or ears of an opponent.

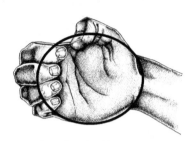

Kumade, or bear hand.

Ippon Nukite

Ippon nukite, or the one-finger spear hand, has the same construction as the flat version of hiraken, except the index finger is extended completely out and its tip is the striking surface. This is not a ready-made weapon but can be used to attack very soft targets such as the eyes.

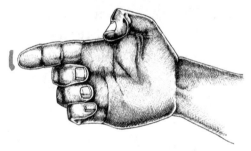

Ippon nukite, or the one-finger spear hand.

Recently, Iain Abernethy[2] has suggested that the extended index finger is rather a guide and that the bent thumb is the actual weapon. The eye attack would then be performed with the thumb in the eye socket, the finger extending along the face pointing toward the ear while the fingers grip the underside of the jaw.

2. http://www.iainabernethy.co.uk/content/practical-kata-bunkai-unsu-ippon-nukite -video

Nihon Nukite

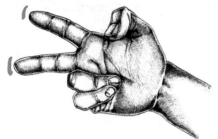

Nihon nukite, or the two-finger spear hand.

Nihon nukite, or the two-finger spear hand, has the same construction as the flat version of hiraken, except the index and middle fingers are extended completely out. It is used to attack the eyes.

Koko

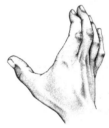

Koko, or tiger's mouth.

Koko, or "tiger's mouth," is formed the same way as hiraken, but with the hand rotated in an ulnar deviation (flat and away from the body) so that the apex of the "V" between the thumb and hand is in line with the radius and ulna. The thumb is still bent. This ready-made weapon is used to strike the Adam's apple.

Shuto

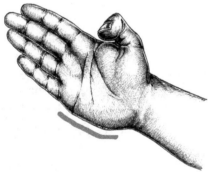

Shuto, or knife hand.

Shuto, or knife hand, is formed by holding the hand straight and flat out from the wrist. The thumb is bent inward. The striking surface is the knife-edge surface of the hand between the little finger and the wrist. It is important to make sure that the fingers are squeezed together tightly to compress the muscles of the hand. This is a ready-made weapon.

Haishu

Haishu, or the backhand, can be configured the same as either shuto or kumade, only this time the striking surface is the back of the hand.

Haito

Haito, or the ridge hand, is the area of the hand between the index finger and wrist. To form this weapon, the thumb is tucked and bent under the hand to expose the correct surface. This ready-made weapon is useful to attack the neck or temple.

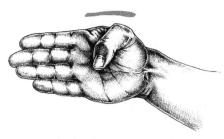

Haito, or ridge hand.

Kakuto

Kakuto, or the bent wrist, is formed by having the hand palm down, then flexing the wrist downward and extending the fingers and thumb to a point. The fingers squeeze together, hardening the tendons and ligaments. The striking surface is the top of the wrist joint.

Kakuto also can be inverted so that the fingers are pointing upward and the wrist brought in line rather than flexed. The fingertips are then the striking surface (normally under the chin), as in the kata Gojushiho Dai.

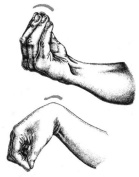

Kakuto, or the bent wrist. Note both the inverted-fingertip striking surface (upper) and the bent-wrist striking surface (lower).

Keito

Keito, or the "chicken head wrist," is formed by making shuto, then bending the wrist to the horizontal plane so that the joint of the thumb that connects it to the hand is facing upward. Next, relax the hand and bend it downward in the horizontal plane (drop the fingers downward). This will expose the top knuckle of the thumb and wrist as the striking surface.

Seiryuto

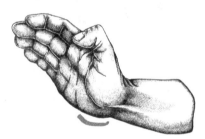

Seiryuto, or the ox jaw hand.

Seiryuto, or the "ox jaw hand," is formed in a way similar to keito. It is formed by making shuto, then supinating the wrist so that the thumb is facing upward. Next, relax the hand and radially deviate it (lift the fingers upward). This will expose the palm-heel edge of the wrist as the striking surface.

Striking Points of the Foot

Like the hand, there are also many parts of the foot that can be used to strike a target. Unlike many of the hand techniques, many of the foot striking surfaces are ready-made weapons.

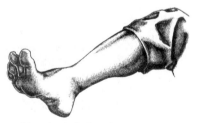

Koshi, or the ball of the foot.

Koshi

Normally the first weapon introduced for the foot is koshi, or the ball of the foot. The ball of the foot is exposed in exactly the same position as when one stands in the tiptoe position. That is, the foot is plantar flexed, and the toes are pulled back. This is a very strong weapon and can be used immediately.

Sokuto

Sokuto, or the blade of the foot, is constructed by dorsiflexing and supinating the foot (pulling it back and turning it outward) and pulling the toes back toward the body. This is similar

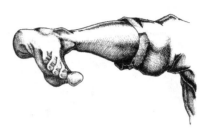

Sokuto, or the blade of the foot.

to standing on the outside edges of the foot. This is often used in side kicks and, depending on which side kick is employed, can slightly change the focus of the kicking weapon. Generally, if yoko geri keage (side snap kick) is employed, the blade edge toward the middle of the foot is used. Likewise, with yoko geri kekomi (side thrust kick), the blade edge toward the heel is used.

Haisoku

Haisoku, or the instep, is constructed by plantar flexing the foot and curling the toes downward. This exposes the instep, which is the striking surface.

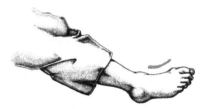

Haisoku, or the instep.

Teisoku

Teisoku, or the sole of the foot, is constructed in the same manner as sokuto, except the sole of the foot is the striking surface. The ability to use the sole comes

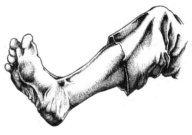

Teisoku, or the sole of the foot.

from the adduction (bringing the leg from outside the body to inside the body) of the femur in the hip joint.

Kakuto

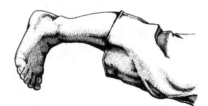

Kakuto, or the heel of the foot.

Kakuto, or the heel of the foot, is constructed by fully dorsiflexing the foot and curling the toes back, exposing the heel. In a back kick position it is important to have the foot pointed downward; however, this position can also be used in a front kick position, where the toes are pointed upward.

Sokusen

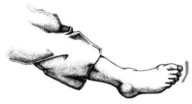

Sokusen, or the toes.

Sokusen, or the toes, can also be used as weapons. For this to be effective, the foot is plantar flexed with the toes straight in front and squeezed together to make a striking surface. This can be used to hit soft parts of the body.

Other Weapons of the Body

In addition to the hands and feet, there are additional weapons that can be used as striking surfaces. Some of these are more devastating since they are harder and closer to the body's center. This is because they are a smaller lever and therefore are more connected to the body. To see this principle at work, have someone stand with their arm in front of them. You will find it easy to push the arm aside by applying pressure to the wrist. But if you push on their elbow, the limb will be much harder to move. Also, the striking surfaces are often more solid compared to the hands and feet.

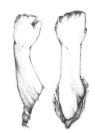

Ude

Ude, the forearms, can be used as weapons. Normally they are in the full supinated or pronated position to tighten the forearm and create a harder and more resilient surface.

Ude, or the forearm.

Empi

Empi, the elbow, is an exceptionally strong weapon. The striking surface can be the front of the elbow or the tip, depending on the angle and direction of the strike. Make sure the wrist is in the fully pronated position so the tendons in the elbow are held tight. In the supinated or relaxed position,

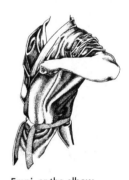

Empi, or the elbow.

the tendons are generally loose and the elbow could be damaged.

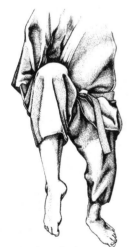

Hittsui

Hittsui, the knee, is another exceptionally strong weapon. It is formed by having the knee in full flexion and the foot in a full plantar flex, with the toes curled under the foot. One common misconception is that the foot should be in a dorsiflexed position; this position relaxes the tendons in the front of the knee and could result in damage to the knee. Only when the foot is in plantar

Hittsui, or the knee.

flexion are these tendons tight, creating a compact, strong weapon used in muay Thai, or Thai boxing.

Others of Note

There are several other striking surfaces used in karate. They include the head, the shoulder, and the hip. These surfaces are hard and solid and are often used in kata, but not in regular practice.

References

Ferrie, E. *Karate-Do: The Way of the Empty Hand.* Ramsbury, UK: Crowood Press, 1996.

Funakoshi, G. *Karate Do Kyohan: Master Text for the Way of the Empty Hand.* San Diego: Neptune Publications, 2005.

Higaonna, M. *Traditional Karate-Do.* Tokyo: Minato Research Publications Co., 1986. Vol. 2, *Performances of the Kata.*

Marieb, E. N., and K. Hoehn. *Human Anatomy and Physiology.* 9th ed. Boston: Pearson, 2012.

Mitchell, D. *Official Karate.* London, Stanley Paul, 1986.

Nakayama, M. *Dynamic Karate: Instruction by the Master.* Tokyo: Kodansha International, 1966.

Nishiyama, H., and R. C. Brown. *Karate: The Art of "Empty-Hand" Fighting.* Boston: Tuttle Publishing, 1960.

Okazaki, T., and M. V. Stricevic. *The Textbook of Modern Karate.* New York: Kodansha International, 1984.

Otsuka, H. *Wado Ryu Karate.* Hong Kong: Masters Publication, 1997.

Pflüger, A. *Karate: Basic Principles.* New York: Sterling, 1967.

Rielly, R. L. *Complete Shotokan Karate: History, Philosophy, and Practice.* Boston: Tuttle Publishing, 1998.

Schmeisser, E. *Advanced Karate-Do.* St. Louis: Focus Publications, 1994.

Yamaguchi, G. *Goju Ryu Karate Kyohan.* Hamilton, ON: Masters Publication, 1999.

CHAPTER 4

Stances, the Body Postures of Karate

Dachi, or stance in karate, is a universal term for body and foot positions, which provide a stable base from which tsuki, uke, keri, and uchi may be executed. In addition, dachi controls body position and distance to the opponent as well as the relative angle between technique and target.

In order to achieve a stable position, the practitioner needs to understand the center of gravity (CG) and its relationship to the base of support. This is covered in depth in the second part of this book. Simply put, the farther apart the feet are and the lower the CG, the more stable the practitioner is. With this concept in mind, it is important to always be cognizant of the position of the body center or CG. We will begin this chapter with a discussion of the main stances. In the next chapter, we will discuss their dynamics and the role of CG in transitioning from one stance to another.

Types of Stances

There are many stances that are used in karate; each one provides a different body position that can be applied to a different scenario. In Okazaki Sensei's book *The Textbook of Modern Karate* (*1*) he describes three major classes of stances. The three classes are natural (shizen tai), fundamental (kihon), and sparring (kumite). Generally, there is good agreement of the stances in most of the readily available literature, and many of the stances are shared between different ryu of karate (*1–10*).

In this classification system there are several major points to consider. The first is the distance of the feet from one another. If the feet are farther apart, such as one and a half to two shoulder widths (as with zenkutsu dachi), the practitioner will be in a lower position, increasing stability. If they are in a higher stance (through the feet being one shoulder width apart, as with renoji dachi), they trade away some balance but then can use gravity to drop into position. These higher stances are often called the "natural" stances.

Along with the height of the center of gravity, the farther apart the feet are, the greater control of distance the practitioner gains with the feet fixed in a single spot. For example, practitioners can transition their body center over a greater distance as they move their body center forward and backward with their feet far apart (e.g., zenkutsu dachi, back to kiba dachi, and then to kokutsu dachi), compared to moving their body center with their feet only a hip width apart (e.g., from renoji dachi, to heiko dachi, and then to teiji dachi).

In addition, stances can be divided into two basic nonexclusive categories according to whether they involve inside or outside tension. This refers to the tension through the stance as the feet connect to the floor. Such tension can have large impacts on the dynamics of transition from one stance to another.

Stances also can be divided according to their posture. While many rely on vertical posture, they can on occasion be on an angle (while maintaining a straight back). The posture must also be considered in relation to the hip position. Generally, there are three major ways to position the hip: front facing (shomen), half front or reverse half front facing (hanmi or gyaku hanmi), and side facing (yoko). A particular stance only allows certain postures. Posture therefore determines what technique can be performed as well as the ways you can transition from one technique to the next. It is for this reason that we are discussing stances and their dynamics early. In short, stances have overarching implications for all techniques.

Quite often, the phrase "heels in line," when talking about a stance with one foot in front of the other, refers to the heels being one directly in front of the other or directly on a line. However, this may be a misconception, and "heels in line" may in fact refer to the heels being on either side of a perpendicular line. This means that when executing kokutsu dachi, or back stance, if the feet were slid toward one another the rear foot would not bump into the back

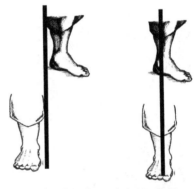

Alignment of the feet in kokutsu dachi. Left: the correct alignment, with the feet placed on either side of a perpendicular line. Right: the less stable variation of the stance, where the heels are directly in line with one another.

heel of the front foot, but rather slide next to it. This would result in the back of the rear heel touching the inside heel of the front foot, which would be more stable. This was described by Mr. Leon Sill, eighth dan ISKF, and makes sense, as it allows the hips the ability to rotate more freely in the hip joint in these stances, provides some additional stability by slightly widening the base of support, and reduces strain on the joints. This is contrary to almost every figure in most published works. Note that in stances where the feet are parallel (such as kiba dachi), heel in line means that the toes and heels are in line with one another.

Natural Stances (Shizen Tai)

The natural stances are generally higher in position than the other two types of stances, and, as their name suggests, are more "natural" types of positions. They are subdivided into three classes: the feet-together stances, the open-leg stances, and the right-angle stances.

Feet-Together Stances

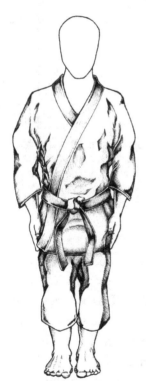

The feet-together stances are frequently used as an attention or beginning stance. However, they can also be used as transition stances due to their fully contracted nature (feet together) and their small radius, which decreases angular momentum and makes any rotation from this position easier to control.

Heisoku Dachi

Heisoku dachi, or formal attention stance, is constructed in a basic sense by having the feet, ankles, and knees together. The knees are straight and the posture from hips to heels is a straight line.

In addition to this configuration, it is also used frequently as a transitional stance where the feet, ankles, and knees are together but with the knees bent as

Heisoku dachi, or formal attention stance.

low as possible without the heels lifting from the floor. This is used as the apex of a contraction during movement and in stepping and rotational movements.

Musubi Dachi

Musubi dachi, or informal attention stance, is constructed by having the ankles and knees together but the feet turned outward to form a ninety-degree angle between the big toes (like a duck). This position is regarded as a little more stable than heisoku dachi and is therefore more frequently used as an attention stance.

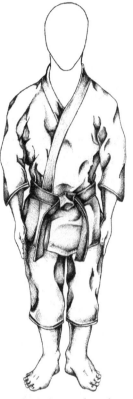

Musubi dachi, or informal attention stance.

Open-Leg and Right-Angle Stances

The open-leg and right-angle stances are truly natural stances. In terms of dynamic feel and shape, they all have their equivalents in the fundamental stances but are executed from a more natural, higher position. The practitioner needs a thorough understanding of the fundamental equivalents to be able to execute these stances correctly.

Another use for these stances is for students who have knee injuries. If a student of mine has a knee injury but has been cleared for light activity by a physician, I often find I can have him or her train by using these stances, since they do not involve the deep knee bends of the kihon dachi. This can allow students to continue training when otherwise they may become discouraged during recovery from an injury.

There are three open-leg stances—hachiji dachi, heiko dachi, and uchi hachiji dachi—and two right-angle stances, renoji dachi and teiji dachi.

Hachiji Dachi

Hachiji dachi, or open-leg stance, is formed by having the feet shoulder width apart with the heels turned inward so the feet point outward. The heels are parallel to the front of the room. (This posture resembles the Japanese character for eight; hachiji dachi literally means "character for eight (八) stance.") The knees are straight, creating a very natural position and easy movement, since the

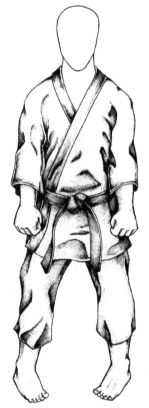

muscles and tendons of the inner thigh are not engaged to the same degree as in heiko or uchi hachiji dachi (see below). The equivalent fundamental stance is shiko dachi, and it is common in Goju-ryu but not so much in Shotokan.

Heiko Dachi

Having the feet shoulder width apart and parallel to the front of the room constructs heiko dachi, or parallel stance. The legs are straight. This stance provides medium connection to the floor by connecting the muscles in the inner thigh, stabilizing the leg laterally to the hip. The equivalent fundamental stance is kiba dachi.

Uchi Hachiji Dachi

Uchi hachiji dachi, or inside natural

Uchi hachiji dachi, or inside natural stance.

Uchi hachiji dachi, or inside natural stance (literally the "upside down character eight (八) stance"), is the opposite of hachiji dachi. It is performed with the legs straight and the feet shoulder width apart parallel to the front of the room. The feet are also turned in with the toes inward and the heels outward. This is the most stable of the three open-leg stances due mainly to the ability to completely engage the *m. satoris* and *m. gracilis* muscles in the front of the hip. There is no fundamental stance equivalent since it is impossible to point the feet inward from a wider position with the feet. However, it is related to Sanchin and Hangetsu dachi, but with an outside tension feel (see next chapter).

Renoji Dachi

Renoji dachi, L stance, or "stand like the character レ stance," is constructed by having the heels in line and the feet about shoulder width in front of one another. The front foot faces forward and the rear foot is pointing outward at a slight angle. The fundamental stance equivalent is zenkutsu dachi. The majority of the weight is on the rear foot as in zenkutsu dachi, where the driving leg is the rear leg.

Teiji Dachi

Teiji dachi, T stance, or "stand like the character 丁 stance," is constructed with the heels in line, one directly behind the other and shoulder width forward. The front forward is pointing directly ahead; the rear is perpendicular to the front. The fundamental stance equivalent is kokutsu dachi.

Fundamental Stances (Kihon Burui)

The fundamental stances are generally performed from a lower position and usually take advantage of at least one knee being fully bent. Having the knee fully bent provides two major advantages: (1) the center of gravity is lowered so the stance is more stable, and (2) the quadriceps (one of the largest muscles in the body) is fully lengthened and ready to contract strongly to straighten the leg.

One important point about bending the knee is to make sure it bends in the same direction the foot points. The knee should always be in line with the foot because the knee joint is a hinge joint and only has at best five degrees of movement laterally before it dislocates out of joint (J. Challis, Penn State University, personal communication). A knee bent off the right angle causes many knee injuries in karate. While the knee has ligaments and tendons to hold it in place before dislocation, continued lateral strain on the knee will cause imbalances and eventually knee issues. Therefore, it is imperative for the practitioner to be cognizant of how the knee is bending at all times and in all movements.

The fundamental stances, due to their low position, are invaluable training stances for three reasons: (1) due to their low position, they develop leg strength, and in the dynamic transitional movements from one to another they develop explosive power. (2) They provide a "perfect" position for the practitioner, which means they provide the strongest position for that base of support. (3) They provide the correct internal "feel," which will in turn allow the practitioner to develop proficiency in the natural stances.

The fundamental stances are divided into two categories depending on the knee's tension. The straddle-leg stances involve outward tension, and the half-moon stances involve inward tension. I discuss the concept of tension in detail later, but it is important to note that the tension can change from inward to outward depending on the needs of the practitioner in that moment in time rather than being tied to a specific stance. Therefore, in some cases inward tension can be exchanged for outward tension within the same stance, so this is a generalization.

Straddle-Leg Stances

The straddle-leg stances have at least one knee bent over the toe. The degree of the bend is directly related to the degree of flexibility of the practitioner's ankle as the practitioner bends the knee until just before the heel lifts from the floor. This can be very hard for practitioners of Western European descent, who tend to have inflexible ankles. In addition, many of these stances are constructed by having a slight outward pressure. That is, the feet are pushing outward and away from the center of the body. This concept will be discussed in detail in the next chapter.

Zenkutsu Dachi

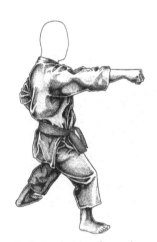

Zenkutsu dachi—forward, front, or "front knee bent stance"—is formed by having the feet one and one half to two shoulder widths in front of each other and separated left to right by one shoulder to one hip distance. Both feet point as far to the front as flexibility allows, and the front knee is bent as far as possible without lifting the heel of the front leg off the floor. The rear leg is straight but not locked or hyperextended. The hips are tucked under the body and can freely move into either hanmi or shomen.

Zenkutsu dachi, or forward stance.

The center of gravity is positioned approximately 60/40 front to back leg and 50/50 laterally. The front ankle is bent strongly, and the knee is over the front toe, similar to the position of a sprinter in the blocks. This places the heel of the front foot almost under the buttock, depending on an individual's femur length. This creates the feeling of dropping the weight and pushing forward.

The rear leg is straight and provides a solid driving connection between the heel of the rear foot and the hip. It is important not to hyperextend or lock the rear leg in place, as this will lift the rear hip and break the lower back posture by lifting the buttock up and backward. This has the effect of removing any drive the rear leg would contribute to the technique since the hip joint would not be seated correctly under the spine.

The feet are one and one half to two shoulder widths apart, depending on flexibility. More specifically, stance length is determined by the farthest distance the feet can be apart and still have the rear heel push weight into the foot with the hips straight (held in shomen). This will vary by age, flexibility, and femur length; however, as long as the 60/40 ratio is met, the front leg is bent, and the rear leg is straight, technically any distance could be considered zenkutsu dachi.

The foot for the front leg is placed so that the outside edge of the foot points straight ahead, although this can be adjusted if one is knock-kneed or bowlegged. This tightens the *m. satoris* and *m. gracilis* muscles and connects the front leg tightly to the hip. The rear foot points as far forward as the practitioner's ankle flexibility allows. It is important not to point the rear foot in such a way as to have to tilt the rear hip upward, destroying the lower back posture. In the dynamic movement of zenkutsu dachi, the rear leg is the driving leg; however, when it is straight, its role changes from driving to providing support as it connects the hip to the torso and to the attacking limb and provides a solid brace for the force that will come back through the body on impact with the target. This is similar to a stick perched at an angle holding up a wall.

The feet are positioned one shoulder width to one hip width apart, and the body weight is positioned equally between the two feet laterally. This gives the stance lateral stability and allows room for the hips to rotate freely. If the stance is too narrow, it loses its lateral stability; if too wide, the front-to-back stability is thrown off due to the heel of the back leg having to connect at an angle to the hip rather than straight behind it.

The overall final construction of this stance provides a strong foundation front to back and reasonable stability side to side. Unfortunately, the weak point of the stance is at the thirty- to forty-five-degree angle to the front, where the rear leg is not aligned to support the body.

An important point to note here is the placement of the front leg of zenkutsu dachi. The position of the knee over the toe, the foot angled slightly inward due to the outside of the edge of the foot being straight, provides a connection through the leg to the hip, with the heel sitting almost directly under the hips. This is universal in all of the fundamental stances. This position is the transitional position for the next move-ment since the quadriceps is fully length-ened, storing much of the potential driving energy for the next movement.

Kiba Dachi

Kiba dachi (straddle or horse-riding stance) is formed by having the feet one and a half to two shoulder lengths apart. The outside edges of the feet are parallel and the knees are bent over the toes in the same construction as the front leg of zenkutsu dachi. The buttocks are tucked so that they line up with the heels when observed from the side.

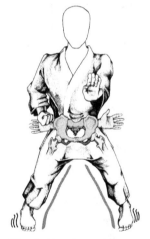

Kiba dachi, or horse-riding stance. Note the outward tension from the hip, which is directly translated to tension on the outsides of the feet.

This stance is very stable and strong in a side-to-side direction but weak in a front-to-back direction. The placement of the legs and feet is important for the strength of this stance. Having the feet parallel, knees bent over the toes, and hips tucked tightens all of the tendons, ligaments, and muscles of the ankle and hip joint into a position that prevents the legs from moving outward (abducted) away from the body.

It is important not to think of the knees as being pushed outward or, worse, to actually do it. Instead, envision a direct connection between the outside edges of the feet and the inside of the hip. The feeling is as if the practitioner is pushing on a flexible bow braced down the inside of the leg and attached to the hip and foot. As the practitioner pushes down, the bow bows outward, creating the bend in the knee. Kiba dachi is formed by two of these bows pushing toward each other, hence the stability of the stance.

There are two main keys to the connection of this stance. First, the outside edges of the feet must be parallel. If they are turned even slightly outward, the tendons, muscles, and ligaments release and allow room for lateral movement in the stance. Second,

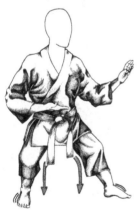

the hip and buttocks must be tucked so they are directly above the ankle when looking from the side. If the buttocks are positioned farther back, there is no way to brace against any force in the stance, and it will inevitably break.

Kokutsu dachi, or back stance. Note the outward tension from the hip of the rear leg. This is directly translated to tension on the outsides of the feet, similar to horse-riding stance, or kiba dachi.

Kokutsu Dachi

Kokutsu dachi, back stance, or "back knee bent stance," is constructed by switching the front leg of zenkutsu dachi to the back leg and angling it at ninety degrees so the outside edge of the back foot is at a right angle to the front. The front foot is one and one half to two shoulder widths directly in front, pointing directly forward, and the leg has a slight bend so it can actively push into the front hip. The buttocks are tucked so the hip is directly in line with the heel of the back foot when viewed from the back. The length of this stance is the same as for zenkutsu dachi and kiba dachi.

The CG is positioned approximately 30/70 with respect to the front and back legs to allow the hips to almost sit over the ankle of the rear leg. This construction creates the strong bow-like pressure in the rear leg, which is the same as kiba dachi. The front leg actively pushes into the hip and back leg to maintain that feeling. An easy way to think about applying pressure in the stance is to actively try to get the feeling of standing on the outside edges of the feet. This maintains the pressure that comes from opening the hips out and provides an outward pressure required by the stance. Another key point is that the front hip must be pushed down as this drives into the rear leg. If the front hip is lifted up, any pressure from the front will lift the practitioner up and over the back leg, breaking the stance. All key points for the positioning of the legs in kiba dachi also hold true for the back leg of kokutsu dachi.

As I said above, this stance is very stable front to back but fairly weak laterally. But this weakness can be offset by thinking about what "heels in line" means. Again, heels in line means they are on either side of an imaginary line rather than on the same line. This slight shift of one to two inches provides a dramatic increase in lateral stability to the stance.

Sochin Dachi (Fudo Dachi)

Sochin dachi (named after the kata Sochin) and fudo (immovable) dachi are sometimes considered the same stance; however, they can have different constructions that are also sometimes interchanged depending on the Shotokan organization. I will define both of them by the more common worldwide designations.

Sochin dachi is constructed with the feet in a place similar to that in zenkutsu dachi (one foot one and one half to two shoulder widths in front of the other and one shoulder width to one hip width apart); however, the actual stance is kiba dachi pushed toward the front in a 60/40 front-to-back weighting. Therefore, both feet point parallel on a thirty-degree angle from the front of the room.

This is a strong stance, weighted forward into a target. It is braced through the construction of the front leg (in the typical bent-knee construction we have discussed previously), with the back leg actively pushing into the front leg. When executing this stance it is important not to let the back leg collapse, but rather keep outward pressure on the outside edge of the foot, which will, in turn, "bow" the leg outward.

Fudo dachi is constructed similarly to kokutsu dachi, except that the weight distribution between the front and back leg is close to 50/50, and the feet are hip distance apart laterally. The front foot points forward. This stance is often used to allow for a strong base to make a block, then to couple translational hip movement to the rotational hip movement for the counterattack as the practitioner transitions from fudo dachi to zenkutsu dachi shomen.

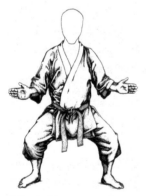

Shiko dachi, or square stance.

Shiko Dachi

Shiko dachi, or square stance, is similar to kiba dachi except that the feet are pointed outward and the knees are able to track over the toes. This allows more free movement in the knee joint, making this stance a more highly mobile version of kiba dachi. Unfortunately, this stance is not commonly used in Shotokan, though it is extensively used in Goju-ryu.

Moto Dachi

Moto dachi, or foundational stance, is derived from zenkutsu dachi except the front foot is moved back the distance of one foot toward the rear leg. This extra movement is then taken up by bending the back leg. Moto dachi represents a foundational kumite stance, and I often refer to it as "neutral" after the neutral position in a stick-shift car. This is because from moto dachi (due to the bends in both legs) it is possible to shift easily to almost any stance.

Half-Moon Stances

The half-moon stances, like the straddle-leg stances, have at least one knee bent over the toe. The difference, however, is that many of these stances are constructed by having a slight inward pressure. That is, the feet are pushing toward the center of the body. Once again, we will discuss this concept more in the next chapter.

Hangetsu Dachi

Hangetsu dachi, or half-moon stance, can be constructed from zenkutsu dachi. In short, the front leg is shifted back toward the back leg by one foot length. The rear leg is turned so the foot points directly toward the front. The front foot is slightly rotated inward so the outside edge of the foot is on a ten- to fifteen-degree angle. Both knees are then bent so they track over the toes, the hips tuck under, and the feet pull inward. There is a drive off the back leg that gives this stance the feeling of pressure that wants to move forward.

One important teaching point is how this inward tension is executed. Too often, it is taught as "pull the knees inward toward each other." This is absolutely wrong and will eventually lead to severe knee injury. The knees are just hinge joints; they extend and flex. There is little or no lateral motion. A better way to instruct

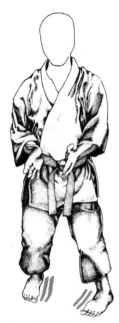

Sanshin dachi, or three battles stance.

students to get the right feel is to tell them to pull the entire leg in between the heels and adductors (inside of the thigh) by squeezing through the hip. The knee is already bent and tracking over the toes, so use the adductors to pull the legs together as if you were standing on a towel on a slippery surface and pulling your legs together from the hip.

Sanchin Dachi

Sanshin dachi, or "three battles stance," is very similar to Hangetsu dachi. It is performed by standing in heiko dachi and bringing one leg directly forward so the feet remain shoulder width apart and the heel of the forward foot is in line with the toes of the rear foot. The front foot is then turned slightly inward to a position similar to Hangetsu, and both knees are bent so that they track over the toes. The practitioner then squeezes the adductors so that there is inward pressure from the inside edge of the feet to the inside of the groin, developing stability in the stance.

Nekoashi Dachi

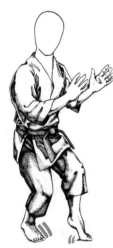

Nekoashi dachi, or cat-foot stance.

Nekoashi dachi, or "cat-foot stance," can be derived from zenkutsu dachi by maintaining the front leg position and swinging the back leg so that it moves to the front. The rear (now front) leg moves forward enough so that 90 percent of the body weight is on the bent leg while 10 percent is on the front. The hip of the weight-bearing leg remains over the heel. The front leg is in a plantar-flexed position so the ball of the foot is touching the floor. The distance between the front and rear legs is dependent on femur length and is normally set in a position such that the shinbone of the front leg is perpendicular to the floor. The legs squeeze inward in a manner similar to what is described above.

Kosa Dachi

In kosa dachi, or "crossing stance," you begin from zenkutsu dachi but then pull the back leg toward the front leg so the shin of the back leg is against the calf of

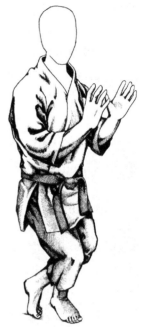

Kosa dachi, or crossing stance.

the front leg. The front foot retains the bent knee position while the back ankle is plantar flexed and the toes are pulled back so that the ball of the foot is in contact with the floor. The hips are tucked under the front leg, and the buttocks are underneath the heel of the front foot. The legs are squeezed together and, along with the straight back and tucked hips, provide stability to the stance.

Sagi Ashi Dachi

The practitioner standing on one leg constructs sagi ashi dachi, or "heron foot stance." The practitioner stands on one leg while the foot of the other leg is most commonly placed so that the instep tucks behind the knee of the standing leg. However, there are other variations, including resting the sole of the foot in the side of the knee of the standing leg. The standing leg can vary between being straight or bent, depending on the purpose, but the most common variation is straight. The legs squeeze together slightly and allow the engagement of the lower abdominals, which provide some stability to the stance.

Sparring Stances (Kumite Burui)

There are equivalent natural stances for each of the fundamental stances. A primary difference between the two classifications is that the fundamental stances represent ideal-world postures used to develop the correct shapes of the positions and how each feels. They allow the practitioner to understand the connection between position and technique. The natural stances require a complete understanding of the fundamental stances in order to be executed correctly. Therefore, the sparring stances represent a compromise between the ideal of technique and the reality of real-time combat.

In addition, the sparring stances are often initiated from a free kamae (posture) position, which in the fundamental world is often

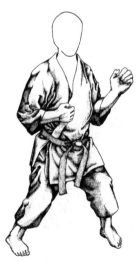

Moto dachi–style kamae.

represented by either moto dachi or renoji dachi. The practitioner then applies tension to the stance, shifting the legs and body center positioning of the individual to the required stance. This is often similar to dropping a cat from a height (not recommended): it will fall and land in an elegant, connected-to-the-floor position from which the cat slinks off.

In this context, the change from a sparring stance to a fundamental or natural stance through the process of executing a technique requires a dynamic change of body weight. For example, the ultimate goal of zenkutsu dachi is to drive the body weight down and forward. The actual posture is only held for a fraction of a second as the technique is delivered. Then the practitioner seamlessly transitions back to the "neutral" position or directly to another stance or position to deliver the next technique. We will discuss this dynamic aspect and the transition between techniques later.

While moto dachi–style kamae is fluid and changing constantly, there are some key points that should be kept in mind. The first is that both knees need to be bent and coiled to allow the practitioner to drive in the direction he or she requires. This means that the weight distribution should be roughly 50/50 between the two legs. Changing between stances, depending on the needs of the situation, is achieved by transferring the bend between the legs. There are trade-offs involved in changing the weight distribution between the two legs. Bending the front leg and transitioning weight to it makes it harder to be swept, and the front leg can also be used to drive forward in a stepping motion. But power from the rear leg for techniques like gyaku zuki or kizami zuki (see below) can be lost. Bending the rear leg positions the body farther away from the opponent and creates additional potential forward drive. However, it is important to note that it can be detrimental to bend the rear leg too far (especially if the femur becomes perpendicular to the ground), as any drive will be in the upward direction rather than in the direction of the opponent. The femur should be held at a thirty- to forty-five-degree angle toward the opponent.

The higher renoji dachi style of kamae loses the bend in the knees and therefore requires the use of gravity and expansion of the hips to drop and drive the technique to work correctly compared to simply using the energy stored through a deep bend in the knees, as in moto dachi. It is important to understand the dynamics of the drop-and-drive type of technique since it is what the practitioner is most likely to face at the beginning of an encounter. Its full dynamics will be discussed in chapter 15. While drop-and-drive dynamics are not often emphasized in regular Shotokan karate practice, they are practiced often in regular training whenever the practitioner moves from a natural stance to a straddle stance.

Finally, the position of the hands is important in kamae. While there are many variations, the most common is a relaxed position, with the elbows close to the body. The forearms and fists point directly to the target (normally the face) like arrows. This removes the need to adjust the angle of the forearms to hit the target with the fist and only requires a simple innervation of the chest and triceps, giving the technique a direct path to the opponent. The angle of the arms changes depending on the distance to the target. If the opponent is some distance away, the forearms will be more parallel to the floor; if the opponent is close, the forearms will be at a much steeper angle. In the first case, with some distance between the combatants, the opponent would have a view of the fist and biceps, but the forearm would be pointing directly at the opponent so he or she would not be able to see it. A common mistake is to have the rear arm hugging the body too much, causing the forearm to point across the opponent. The rear hand must point at the opponent before the technique can be thrown. Otherwise, you would need multiple trajectories to hit the opponent, thus slowing down the technique. Additionally, by having the elbows close to the body, they can be immediately connected to the body and rotated as a single unit for blocking.

Conclusion

The many stances of karate serve a wide variety of purposes. They are not rigidly fixed but represent ways to use body weight effectively, taking into account both the distance between the body center and the opponent as well as the rotational position of the body relative to the opponent. In addition, they provide the bracing required to give the best body alignment for techniques by connecting the body to the floor.

Notes

1. T. Okazaki and M. V. Stricevic, *The Textbook of Modern Karate* (New York: Kodansha International, 1984).
2. H. I. Cho, *The Complete Tae Kwon Do Hyung* (Los Angeles: Unique Publications, 1989).
3. G. Funakoshi, *Karate Do Kyohan: Master Text for the Way of the Empty Hand*. (San Diego: Neptune Publications, 2005).
4. M. Higaonna, *Traditional Karate-Do* (Tokyo, Japan: Minato Research Publications Co., 1986), Vol. 5(2), *Performances of the Kata*.
5. H. Kanazawa, *Black Belt Karate: The Intensive Course* (Tokyo: Kodansha International, 2006).
6. M. Nakayama, *Dynamic Karate: Instruction by the Master* (Tokyo: Kodansha International, 1966), 308.
7. H. Nishiyama and R. C. Brown, *Karate: The Art of "Empty-Hand" Fighting* (Boston: Tuttle Publishing, 1960).
8. H. Otsuka, *Wado Ryu Karate* (Hong Kong: Masters Publication, 1997).
9. S. Toguchi, *Okinawan Goju-Ryu: The Fundamentals of Shorei-Kan Karate* (Burbank, CA: Ohara Publications, 1976), 191.
10. G. Yamaguchi, *Goju Ryu Karate Do Kyohan* (Hamilton, ON: Masters Publication, 1999).

CHAPTER 5

The Dynamics of Stances

Dachi, or stances, as previously discussed, provide a connection between the practitioner and the ground. This connection is essential for the proper execution of karate techniques such as tsuki, uchi, keri, and uke. The stances of karate are the strongest possible positions for the execution of techniques. They also provide reinforcement for absorbing the reaction force generated by the body when it comes into contact with the target.

To make proper use of stances, the practitioner needs to be aware that a stance is much more than a set leg and body position. It is more a dynamic relationship with the floor that allows quick movement through the use of ground reaction force. Therefore, it is important to consider the dynamics of stances both in the static final positions as well as dynamically during movement. A strong dynamic stance requires proper weight distribution, foot position and connection to the floor, leg tension, and hip position and tension. One must also understand how these factors relate to the static stance as well as to dynamic movement.

This chapter will discuss the dynamics of stances in both static and dynamic settings. In addition, we will look at how stance dynamics relate to other aspects of karate.

Stance Tension

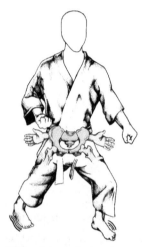

Forward stance in the half-face hip position (zenkutsu dachi hanmi), an example of outward tension. Note that the tension is on the outside edges of the feet; this tension originates from opening the hips outward.

In karate there are two major types of stances. They are differentiated based on the direction of tension to the floor and can be either inside (uchi ni shime) or outside (soto ni shime). In outside-tension stances, the tension in the stance pushes away from the body center. This is felt when the feet have slight pressure on the floor in a direction that is away from the body center. For example, if the practitioner were standing in slippery socks, his or her feet would split outward based on the tension (see first illustration in this section). The opposite is true of the other stance type, inward tension. For inward tension, the feet feel as if they are pulling together (see second illustration in this section). For example, if the practitioner were again standing in slippery socks, his or her feet would slide together toward the body center.

Slight tension in the stance plays several crucial roles. First, the dynamic connection between the feet and the floor allows the practitioner to grip the floor more strongly and stabilizes the stance. Second, the dynamics of the stance allow quick movement, as the practitioner just needs to relax the stance to begin moving to the next position. Third, tension keeps the stance active throughout the movement, allowing the body to connect to the floor and providing a feeling of directionality in the technique.

It is important to note that the tension does not in any way come from the knees. The tension is created from a relationship between the inward tension and outward tension of the foot, on the one hand, and the inside tension and outside tension of the hip and upper thigh. The knees are simply bent to some degree over the toe depending on the stance. Any lateral tension on the knee is very dangerous and will damage the knee joint over time.

In addition, the feeling of tension with the floor should not be excessive. The feeling is just to connect the foot to the floor and provide adequate pressure to let the practitioner push off it. If there is excessive pressure, two things will happen: (1) the upper hip will lock up, preventing fluid hip motion, and (2) the practitioner's hips will rise upward as the tension increases (like squeezing a tube of toothpaste, it will overflow).

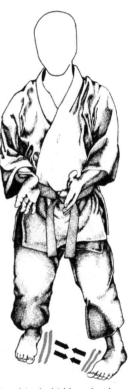

Sanchin dachi (three battles stance), an example of inside tension. Note the knees bending over the toes and the feet pulling inward. The tension originates from the hips pulling inward.

Examples of outside-tension stances include many of the fundamental stances such as the straddle-leg stances discussed in the previous chapter, including zenkutsu dachi, kiba dachi, kokutsu dachi, and others. Inside-tension stances are the half-moon stances discussed previously, including Hangetsu dachi, sanshin dachi, and nekoashi dachi. It is interesting to note that full-length fundamental stances such as zenkutsu dachi are generally outside-tension stances, while shorter-length fundamental stances such as hangestu dachi are inside-tension stances.

Shime

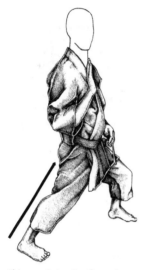

Shime, originating from the floor through the drive of the back leg and setting the limb under the hip, driving the body center forward.

The concept of shime was initially introduced to me by Dr. David Hooper (fourth dan, JKA) and Mr. Steve Ubl (eighth dan, WTKO). Shime refers to the leg's connection to the hip. The example Dr. Hooper gave me involved the back leg of zenkutsu dachi and how it should be pushing the back hip inward and upward toward the spine (D. Hooper, personal communication). If done correctly, the buttocks are tucked underneath the spine and the gluteus muscles are flexed, producing a straight lower back. This upward pressure from the floor through the leg is referred to as shime and provides the basis of inward and outward tension. Generally speaking, outward pressure has both legs pushing in toward the body center by grabbing the floor and pushing toward it. It could be envisioned as pushing against a brick wall that is toppling toward you. Outside-tension shime is a little different. This time you are pulling your legs toward your body center, similar to holding up a wall that is falling away from you. This connection to the hip is vital.

Stance Connection and Foot Tension

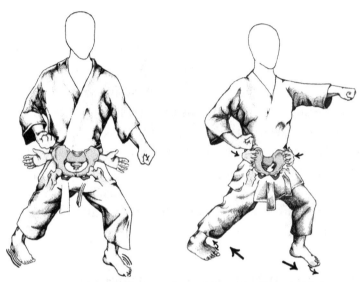

Change in tension through the feet in forward stance (zenkutsu dachi) that results in changing the hip position between hanmi and shomen. Left picture: hips in the half face of hanmi position. Notice the tension through the outside edges of the feet originating from the hip being opened wide. Right picture: hips in shomen resulting in a change in tension from the outside edges of the feet to the feet pushing away from one another in an outward direction. This change in foot tension results in the hips contracting, resulting in the rotational movement of the hips from a half- to front-facing position.

Much of the tension in the stance should be derived from the way the feet are connected to the floor. In zenkutsu dachi hanmi, for example, the feet are pushing outward from the outside edges of the feet on an approximately thirty-degree angle away from the body. In shomen, the stance tension changes to the toes of the front foot and heels of the back foot pushing away from one another. Interestingly, this tension can be changed significantly depending on the needs of the stance. For example, in shomen the tension can be changed to inside tension, with both the front and rear feet pulling inward. In addition, if the hips need to be fully turned to shomen in zenkutsu dachi and the feet are in line, this can be achieved by changing to inward tension by pulling the inside edges of the feet inward.

For inside-tension stances, the feet are generally pulled inward with additional pressure in the inside of the foot. This allows for the correct hip and leg tension set up for the stance.

It is important to note that while one would stand on the inside or outside edges of the foot, this is in feeling only. The entire foot is always connected to the floor; only the pressure changes depending on the stance. The concept is similar to standing on a Dr. Scholl's kiosk at Walmart, where foot pressure is measured and recorded as a heat map. Sometimes these machines were used to experiment with different stances and make sure inside and outside foot tension was correct.

Tension and How It Relates to Dynamic Movement

Inside and outside tension is critical to movement from stance to stance. This concept is discussed in detail in chapter 17; however, a brief introduction is provided here.

Quickly being able to alter the dynamic tension in the stance from foot to hip is key to executing techniques in quick succession and, moreover, moving from one position to another quickly and efficiently. If we take the movement of stepping forward from zenkutsu dachi hanmi to zenkutsu dachi hanmi and then rotating to shomen zenkutsu dachi as an example, it is a clear dynamic movement of outside to inside to outside tensions.

Before the step, the zenkutsu dachi hanmi is an outside-tension stance, with the feet pushing outward on the outside edges of the feet. The movement is then initiated by the feet changing to inside tension (pulling through the heel and toes of the feet toward the body center), which rotates the hip. It could also be argued that it is the hips that initiate the tension change in the feet. The feet again initiate movement, traversing through heisoku dachi, which is an inside-tension stance. The legs use the momentum gained from the inside tension to continue swinging the back leg through to the front, at which time the front (now rear) leg engages, switches to outside tension, and drives the body forward. The front foot grabs the floor, connecting the stance in an outside-tension feel with the feeling of standing on the outside edges of the feet. The front foot grabs the floor, creating a feeling of outside tension as well as a feeling of standing on the outside edges of the feet. The movement is completed by squeezing the hips and changing the tension in the feet from pushing on the outside edges to pushing away from the body center through the toes of the front leg and heel from the back leg. This allows the change in the hips from hanmi to shomen.

These concepts are especially important with respect to the change from outside- to inside-tension stances and are one thing that Shotokan practitioners do not generally practice enough. There is a lot of practice changing position from outside- to outside-tension stances but not enough from outside to inside and vice versa. It is useful to practice drills that have you step freely from zenkutsu dachi, to nekoashi dachi, to kiba dachi, and to hangestu dachi. Gaining proficiency in this allows you to connect the stance better in the shorter in-between movements of the fundamental half-moon stances. This in turn teaches better muscle memory in developing the ability to connect one's body to the floor on demand during kumite.

References

Higaonna, M. *Traditional Karate-Do*. Tokyo: Minato Research Publications Co., 1986. Vol. 5(2), *Performances of the Kata*.

Nakayama, M. *Dynamic Karate: Instruction by the Master*. Tokyo: Kodansha International, 1966.

Nishiyama, H., and R. C. Brown. *Karate: The Art of "Empty-Hand" Fighting*. Boston: Tuttle Publishing, 1960.

Okazaki, T., and M. V. Stricevic. *The Textbook of Modern Karate*. New York: Kodansha International, 1984.

Otsuka, H. *Wado Ryu Karate*. Hong Kong: Masters Publication, 1997.

Pflüger, A. *Karate: Basic Principles*. New York: Sterling, 1967.

Rielly, R. L. *Karate Training: The Samurai Legacy and Modern Practice*. Rutland, VT: Tuttle Publishing, 1985.

Schmeisser, E. *Advanced Karate-Do*. St. Louis: Focus Publications, 1994.

Toguchi, S. *Okinawan Goju-Ryu: The Fundamentals of Shorei-Kan Karate*. Burbank, CA: Ohara Publications, 1976.

Yamaguchi, G. *Goju Ryu Karate Do Kyohan*. Hamilton, ON: Masters Publication, 1999.

CHAPTER 6

Tsuki: Thrusting Techniques

Tsuki is a class of karate hand techniques often regarded as synonymous with punching. However, this class of technique is actually far broader and is more accurately described as a set of thrusting techniques. They involve the path the hand travels to the target relative to the long bone of the forearm (*1*). That path is relatively direct to the target (moving parallel to the forearm), and the striking surface is at the end of the forearm.

Principles of Tsuki

There are three principles important for executing tsuki correctly. The first is that the elbow of the striking limb rubs close to the side of the body until the elbow passes the torso. This is universal for all tsuki, and it could be said that the differentiation in the path of any tsuki technique only occurs once the elbow passes the body. This ensures that the correct muscles in the shoulder, chest, and back are connected to the technique as it accelerates from the hip. It is good to imagine performing all tsuki hitting the imaginary target with the point of the elbow and the forearm (and thus the striking surface, such as the fist, just gets in the way).

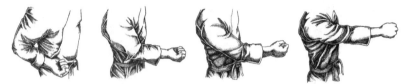

Path of the straight punch, or choku zuki.

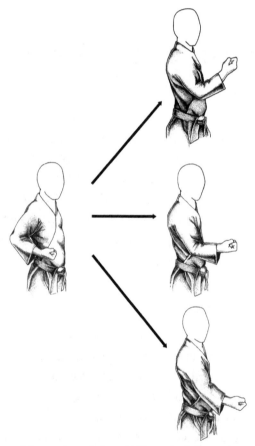

Targeting of the straight punch, or choku zuki. The path of the punch is set when the elbow passes the body as the punch is executed to the face, jodan (top); the stomach, chudan (middle); and the groin, gedan (bottom).

With this concept in mind, it is important to have the forearm on its correct path to the target in terms of level (jodan is face level, chudan is stomach level, and gedan is groin level) before the elbow leaves the side of the body. The simplest way to imagine this is if the forearm, from fist to elbow, is pointing like an arrow at the target by the time the elbow leaves the body. This ensures the correct and most direct path to the target. The "aiming" should be done with natural motion. For example, there is no need to unduly stress the biceps when aiming at jodan, as this will slow the course of the technique. Rather, think of the movement as being as natural as reaching for a glass in an eye-level cabinet.

The second principle refers to the fist of the striking hand on the hip at the beginning and during the initiation of the technique. In particular, the radius and ulna need to be rotated fully so that the thumb is twisted as far to the outside of the body as possible. If the right hand is on the hip, the hand is rotated as far clockwise as possible. This tension needs to be maintained at least until the elbow passes the torso, but preferably until the moment of contact with the target. This ensures that the elbow is tight to the body through the initial stages of the technique. It can also be advantageous to twist the forearm a little tighter as the technique is executed. This will allow a sharper rotation at the conclusion of the technique.

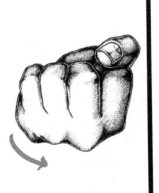

Side of Body

Correct position for the fist in the preparatory position before the execution of a thrusting technique.

The third major principle is to only contract the muscles that drive the forward motion of the technique while relaxing all others. This means concentrating on contracting only the muscles that move the body center forward

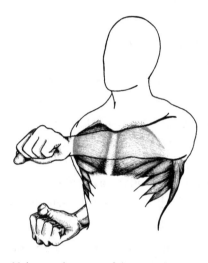

Major muscle groups of the torso that need to be employed at the conclusion of choku zuki.

and those that drive the limb forward. In choku zuki, the only upper-body muscles that need to contract during the movement are the chest and triceps.

In addition, at the conclusion of the technique it is important to have the striking limb in the correct position to be able to lock it down for the split second of impact. You do this by contracting the *pectoralis* muscles in the chest and the *latissimus dorsi* muscles of the back equally, while letting the shoulders relax. This ensures that the striking limb is connected strongly to the body at the moment of impact. If the arm is too far extended, the back cannot be engaged. Likewise, if the arm is not extended enough, the chest is not engaged. If the shoulder is lifted, it will not be able to set in the socket and the arm will be disconnected from the rest of the body, causing the punch to lose much of the accompanying body mass. The resulting impact will be severely reduced. An easy way to assess the correct position is to extend both arms in front of the body at a ninety-degree angle to the torso, while pushing the shoulders down. Next, dorsiflex the hands at the wrist; this should result in the palm heels of the hands pointing upward. Finally, rotate the hands outward and down so that the fingers are pointing at the floor. This position, if the arms are fully extended, with the shoulders pushing down and the fingers pointing down, is the correct position. Both the back and chest muscles should be engaged. This should result in a feeling of a ball or an empty space in the armpit. When keeping this position, the elbow points to the floor.

The radius and ulna are free to rotate as needed while keeping the upper arm (humerus) locked in position.

Types of Tsuki

Tsuki can be broadly divided into two major categories. The first is composed of one-handed tsuki, where a single hand strikes the opponent. The second includes two-handed tsuki, where both hands strike the opponent (*2–4*).

One-Handed Tsuki

There are two major positions for one-handed tsuki. The first is where the tsuki hand is on the same side as the leading leg (e.g., the right hand is punching and the right leg is forward). There are two or possibly three terms describing different aspects of this. The first is jun, which means that the legs are stationary and the same-side leg and hand are out. The second is oi, or lunge, and is when the same leg is moving forward while the tsuki is being executed. There is arguably a third called kizami, which refers to the difference in hip position. Oi and jun are executed from a shomen, or front-facing hip position, while kizami is executed from a hanmi, or half-face hip position.

The second major position for one-handed tsuki is gyaku, which refers to when the tsuki hand is opposite or reverse to the leg that is out (e.g., the left hand punching with the right leg forward). Due to its nature, it is always performed in shomen. There is no distinction between stepping and nonstepping forms of gyaku zuki.

One other important point is the position of the opposite or retracting hand. For beginners, the hand should be rotated immediately and drawn tightly and sharply back to the hip. This principle, hikite, helps balance the torso muscles across the body during the execution of the technique. As the practitioner advances, and provided he has an understanding of what muscles need to contract, the full motion becomes less important; however, the feeling of this contraction in the opposite hand must always be present.

Finally, the timing of the technique is vital for hitting the target with the entire body rather than just the momentum of the arm. This means that the body center needs to be in motion toward the target at the moment of impact and not stopped before impact. Initially, this is taught in terms of correct hand and foot timing. But it can be argued that as long as the hip is in motion, the technique can hit at any point. This will be discussed later.

In total, there are approximately seven different one-handed tsuki. All of them have the aforementioned principles in common. The elbow is positioned tightly against the body until it passes the torso. The wrist is fully rotated in the opposite direction and released at the moment of impact. And, finally, all muscles except those engaged with the forward motion should be completely relaxed until the moment of impact. At this instant, the muscles of the back and shoulder are connected to lock the technique down.

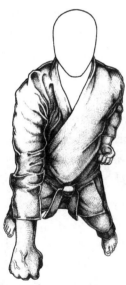

Choku zuki, or the straight punch.

Choku Zuki—Straight Punch

Choku zuki is the "bread and butter" technique of Shotokan. It takes a direct, complete, and straight path from hip to target. The radius and ulna are maximally rotated so that the fist is also completely rotated over. The palm is down and the arm is straight but not locked so that the radius and ulna are in a straight line with the humerus. The hips are in a final shomen position and directly under the torso so that the driving leg can connect correctly to the floor. The technique may be executed from either jun or gyaku.

Tate Zuki—Vertical Punch

Tate zuki follows the same path as choku zuki, except the elbow stops one fist width beyond the torso and the fist is rotated halfway so that the palm is facing toward the body. This is a short-range punch, but due to a fairly long path that allows momentum to build and the close connection to the body through the elbow, it is very powerful.

Kizami Zuki—Thrust Punch

Kizami zuki is a straight punch that is executed in a fashion similar to choku zuki, but the hips are rotated to a hanmi position once the elbow passes the torso. This extends the reach of the technique, but it is less connected to the body due to its extension. Often, kizami zuki is executed by the front hand in a fully relaxed fashion from kamae. It is important to remember to only innervate the muscles that are required for the punch and not to overextend the technique so

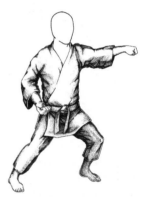

Kizami zuki, or the thrust punch.

that the chest becomes stretched out. In addition, it is common to see people lean forward from the chest and shoulder to cover distance. This has the effect of pushing the hip backward, thereby losing the drive from the rear leg and effectively breaking the connection of the hip to the floor. The illustrations accompanying the next technique, age zuki, offer a clear demonstration of this.

Age Zuki—Rising Punch

Age zuki takes a rising path toward the target. Once the elbow passes the torso, the punch rises from an initial chudan (stomach) trajectory as the elbow leaves the body to a jodan (face) trajectory.

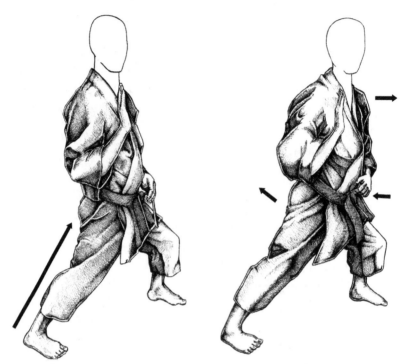

Examples of good (left) and poor (right) body position in the execution of tsuki. Notice the correct use of shime in the left picture. This allows the driving leg to correctly seat under the hips, thus driving the body center forward. However, in the right picture, the body leans forward, which causes the rear of the hip to lift, not allowing the leg to seat correctly under the hip. This causes the body center to shift backward, away from the target, resulting in a loss of power in the technique.

The overall effect is that the arm scoops upward. This technique therefore strikes both upward and into the target simultaneously and is ideal for hitting under the chin or philtrum under the nose.

Mawashi Zuki—Round Punch

Mawashi zuki takes an outside to inside path to the target. This will strike the target at approximately a thirty-degree angle from the center and is designed to get around a front guard and hit the side of the jaw squarely at an angle from ear to chin. This technique is achieved by initiating the rotation of the fist after the elbow passes the torso.

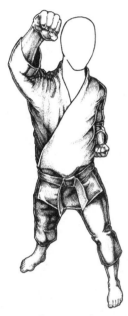

Mawashi zuki, or the round punch.

This has the effect of releasing the elbow early compared to choku zuki (where the elbow is kept in the straight line throughout the technique) and allowing it to take the round path.

Kagi Zuki—Hook Punch

Kagi zuki, or hook punch, has a final position of ninety degrees with the elbow in the same position as choku zuki, but the forearm is at ninety degrees facing inward. It is executed by passing the elbow close and tight to the body and, once past, keeping the elbow on the same straight, forward trajectory while the radius and ulna rotate sharply. This has the effect of snapping the forearm to a ninety-degree angle. It is important not to release the elbow early as is often observed in tournament Heian godan. Keep it tight until the elbow passes the torso. Also, rotate the radius and ulna tightly; this will result in the fist being slightly over-rotated in the final technique. A good check for the final position of the technique is to extend the forearm while holding the rest of the body still. This should result in a perfect final position for choku zuki.

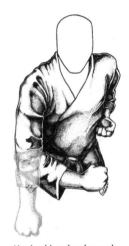

Kagi zuki, or hook punch. Note that the final elbow position is the same as a finished straight punch, or choku zuki. Therefore, in both punches the elbow follows an identical path.

Ura Zuki—Close Punch

Ura zuki is a very close-ranged punch. Its final position has the elbow still touching the torso and the fist still fully rotated in its initial palm-upward position. It is effectively the initial movement of every tsuki that we have discussed here.

Two-Handed Tsuki

The second major class of tsuki is where both hands are employed to strike the target simultaneously. All of the three principles previously discussed also hold true for these techniques (*2–4*).

Yama Zuki—Mountain Punch

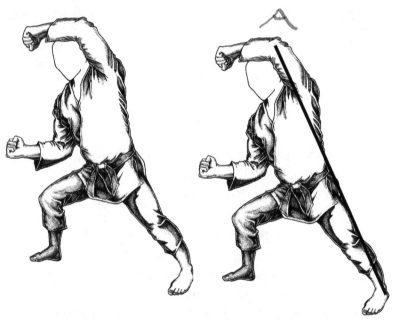

Yama zuki, or mountain punch. The heel of the left leg to the elbow of the upper arm forms a straight line to the floor. This line is on an angle toward the target. Note that the back is still straight.

Yama zuki is performed from the hanmi position (hips facing half forward) and is effectively mawashi zuki (round punch, the upper arm) and ura zuki (close punch, lower arm). Both fists are vertically in line and directly above and below each other. It is executed with a slight lean in the stance so that from the elbow of the mawashi zuki to the heel of the extended support leg is a single line. Yama zuki gets its name for two reasons. The first is the position of the elbow in the mawashi zuki, which represents the peak of a mountain. The second is that with the head and two arms extended above and below, the technique looks like the Japanese kanji for yama (山), or mountain.

Awase Zuki—U Punch

Awase zuki is a slightly toned-down version of yama zuki. It can be executed from the shomen position and has the gyaku hand in an extended ura zuki and the jun hand in a choku zuki position. Awase zuki can also be shortened so that the ura zuki is in the correct position and the choku zuki is shortened. If it is executed from the hanmi position, both techniques can be executed at the correct lengths.

Heiko Zuki—Parallel Punch

Heiko zuki is two choku zuki executed simultaneously. They are normally executed from the shomen position.

Hasami Zuki

Hasami zuki is two mawashi zuki executed simultaneously. Once again, they are normally executed from the shomen position. This is used in the kata Chinte.

Variations on the Striking Weapon

Any of these tsuki can be executed with any hand technique that is reinforced in the same direction as the forearm. This opens up a wide variety of weapons to the karateka. Often these techniques are practiced with seiken, or the front two knuckles of the fist.

However, many other options are available, including ippon-ken (single extended knuckle), hiraken (extended fist—second joint is used to strike), taisho (palm heel), and nukite (finger tips). With nukite, tate (vertical finger tips), nihon (two finger tips), or ippon (single finger tip) can be used.

Notes

1. E. Schmeisser, *Advanced Karate-Do* (St. Louis: Focus Publications, 1994).
2. M. Nakayama, *Dynamic Karate: Instruction by the Master* (Tokyo: Kodansha International, 1966), 308.
3. H. Nishiyama and R. C. Brown, *Karate: The Art of "Empty-Hand" Fighting* (Boston: Tuttle Publishing, 1960).
4. T. Okazaki and M. V. Stricevic, *The Textbook of Modern Karate* (New York: Kodansha International, 1984).

CHAPTER 7

Keri: Kicking Techniques

One difference between martial arts styles developed in Asia and many of the Western arts is the refinement of the legs and feet as striking weapons. In Shotokan karate in particular, kicking techniques, or keri, are seamlessly integrated into the curriculum and are one of the six major classes of techniques (tsuki, uke, uchi, nage, keri, and dachi).

Keri does have some advantages compared with techniques executed with the arms. Specifically, they have a longer reach since the legs are longer than the arms and they are generally more powerful, since the legs contain more muscle mass compared to the arms. Finally, in self-defense situations, the attacker can be surprised by the use of the legs in combat. Along with these advantages, there are also some drawbacks. First, the balance is diminished since the body is only supported on one leg. Additionally, kicks can be slower and less coordinated than arm techniques, since the legs are not used for fine movement, as the arms and hands are.

In Shotokan, kicking techniques are practiced above the head (similar to taekwondo). This is contrary to many Okinawan karate and grounded Chinese styles of martial arts that do not kick above the waist. The argument for low kicks is made in terms of minimizing the time the kicker is standing on a single leg and reducing the chance that the kicking leg may be grabbed. However, in Shotokan, high kicks are used as a training aid to develop legs and muscles that connect to the hip. Similarly, the lower straddle-leg stances are training aids for the much looser free kamae stances.

Important Points in Kicking

The first major teaching point for kicking is the preparative knee lift. It is vital that the leg be quickly drawn high and tight and that the femur be at least parallel to the floor. This allows the correct path of the limb to the target with minimal torque to the knee. In addition, it is important that the extending limb retract along the same path back to the initial load position.

The second major point in kicking is to closely monitor the path of the kick. The path should be effortless and allow correct movement through the hip joints of both legs and correct extension of the knee joint. There should be no lateral movement. The leg should extend and retract naturally along the same path. To achieve this, it is important to practice the kick slowly and in a controlled fashion. This will help develop the correct stabilizing muscles as well as reinforce the correct neuromuscular pathways to fire the muscles in the correct sequence.

The third major point is to pay very close attention to the supporting leg. At least half the drive of the kick is derived from this leg, since it is in direct contact with the ground and should (as in almost any technique) contribute a significant portion of the forward drive. It must be rotated or set into the correct position to provide the maximal drive, from floor to hip, and be precisely timed with the impact. The position of the supporting leg will vary according to the direction of the kick and the type of kick, whether keage or kekomi (see chapter 18).

The fourth major point is to make sure the correct weapon is exposed to the target and at the correct angle. If the wrong weapon hits, not only could the kick be ineffectual or off balance, it may indicate that the path and final position of the kick is incorrect. One example is in the side snap kick (see below), where the hip must be turned over enough so that the leg correctly rotates in the hip. Otherwise, the impact will be taken on the little toe rather than on the blade of the foot.

The fifth major point is to avoid hyperextending the leg. Keep the joints soft; that is, make sure the joints are not hyperextended at the full extension of the kick. Repeated jarring through hyper-extension of the kick will inevitably lead to injury.

Finally, it is important to develop flexibility and only kick within the limits of your flexibility. Flexibility in this context does not mean how high the leg can be swung, but rather how high the leg can be lifted with control. It is this balance of strength and flexibility that will allow the correct mix of body alignment and force for the impact of the kick while keeping the kicker injury free.

Types of Kicks

Kicks in karate can be divided into four major classes, from which all kicks can then be derived. The first class are the mae, or front kicks; the second are the yoko, or side kicks; the third are the mawashi, or turning kicks (sometime also called roundhouse kicks); and the last are the ushiro, or back kicks.

Front Kicks

Front kicks take a vector from the front of the body straight to the opponent, as if you were pointing directly ahead.

Mae Geri

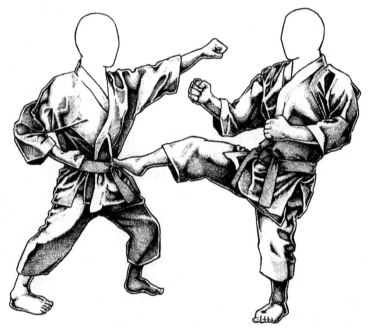

Mae geri, or front kick.

The front kick, mae geri, moves in a direct diagonal line from the floor to the target. It can be performed from either the front or back leg and may be either keage (snap) or kekomi (thrust). Key points for the kick are to lift the leg high and tight in the preparatory position, and during the retraction to bring the ankle as close to the buttocks as possible. The foot is pulled back at the ankle (dorsiflexion), with the toes also pulled back. The leg then extends toward the target, and the foot is extended (plantar flexion) and the toes are pulled back so that the ball of the foot makes contact with the target. Note that the ankle goes from dorsiflexion to plantar flexion during the extension of the leg (basically, the foot is kept level as it moves toward the target). The trajectory of the ankle and foot to the target is a straight line. This can be demonstrated by stretching a belt, or obi, from the heel of the back foot (kicking leg) to the target; as the leg moves, the ankle moves along this line. The hips at the point of contact contract slightly upward and are in the shomen position. The hips at the beginning may be in either hanmi or shomen. If they start in hanmi, then they rotate and tuck; if in shomen, they just tuck.

The support leg drives into the technique and has the effect of pushing the body center into the target. As with all techniques, the drive of the hip through the grounded leg must be timed to the impact of the technique. That is, the hip must still be in motion toward the target as the foot hits the target, otherwise only the weight of the kicking leg will be transferred to the target, as compared to the entire body.

Variations on Mae Geri

Kin Geri

Kin geri, or groin kick, is executed in exactly the same way as mae geri keage, or front snap kick, except for that the foot remains in plantar flexion throughout the kick and the weapon is the instep. The path of the kick is an upward swing and is ideal for hitting the groin.

Mikazuki Geri

Mikazuki geri, or crescent kick, starts from a hanmi (half front face) position, forward stance (zenkutsu dachi), or horse-riding stance (kiba dachi). The leg initiates the movement directly across the body toward the target, similar to a sideways mae geri; however,

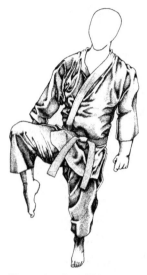

Hiza geri, or knee kick. Note that the final foot position is planar flexed.

the hips are rotated only once the preparatory position is reached. This has the effect of creating a horizontal arc to the kick. The striking weapon is the sole of the foot, which is dorsiflexed and rotated inward. This technique is seen in the Shotokan kata movement #15 in Heian godan or movement #28 in Bassai Dai in *Best Karate* by M. Nakayama (see under references).

Hiza Geri

Hiza geri, or knee kick, is simply the preparatory position of mae geri. The hips are fully extended, pushed inward, and tilted upward, similar to the final position of mae geri. The foot is plantar flexed to increase stability in the striking knee.

Kiri Geri

Kiri geri, or cutting kick, is halfway between the roundhouse kick (mawashi geri) and front kick (mae geri). In execution it is very similar to mae geri, but instead of initiating the kick perpendicular to the floor, the kick is loaded so that the shin is at a thirty-degree angle to the floor, with the ankle to the outside of the body and the knee at the center of the body. This gives the kick an angle that is ideal for hitting a surface that is not square to the kicker, as with an opponent in the hanmi, or side-facing position.

Gyaku Mawashi Geri

This kick is related more to kiri geri than to mawashi geri. In short, it is simply kiri geri in reverse. This time the hips are fully extended into a reverse half-facing position (gyaku hanmi), and the load is at the opposite thirty-degree angle to kiri, with the knee at the center and the ankle on the opposite side of the body. The kick then twists inward toward the opponent.

It is important to note that for all of these kicks the knee has no lateral motion but simply extends naturally straight out toward the target. The angle is set up by the femur rotating longitudinally relative to the hip.

Mae Tobi Geri

There are two common versions of mae tobi geri, or jumping front kick. The first is a straight jump and kick off the front leg. The second is a scissor motion, where the back knee lifts and the other leg does the kick. This can be extended into nidan tobi geri, where both the back and the front leg kick during the jump.

Side Kicks

Side kicks, or yoko geri, are generally performed with the opponent to the side. The striking surface is the blade or side edge of the foot. To achieve this position, the foot is dorsiflexed toward the shin and the toes are pulled inward. The foot is rotated laterally to a plantar-flex position, exposing the blade of the foot.

Yoko Geri Keage

Yoko geri keage, or side snap kick, is designed to stop the opponent in their tracks. It does so by concentrating on a strong, very sharp retraction and hits the target on an approximately forty-five degree upward vector. The preparatory position has the knee lifted upward so that the femur is at least parallel to the floor and outward, similar to a cobbler stretch. I tell my students to imagine that their heel runs up a curtain rail running along the inside of

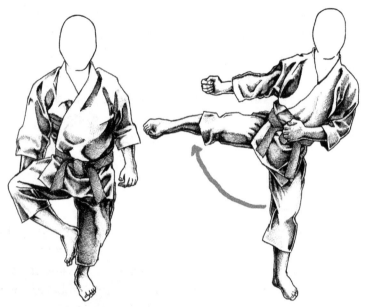

Yoko geri keage, or side snap kick. The preparatory position is shown on the left, and the final kick position is shown on the right. The foot moves through a forty-five-degree upward vector to the target as the hips drive toward the target.

their supporting leg. Once in this position, the leg simply straightens naturally along a line from hip to heel. Rotating and pushing the hip of the supporting leg into the target achieves the upward arc to the kick, and this is the most important concept of the kick. This rotation and pushing of the hip has the effect of moving the body center toward the target and must be timed so that the hip is still driving toward the target as the foot impacts the target. There should be no time during the execution of the kick when the knee of the kicking leg torques laterally or is lower than the ankle. The supporting foot should not need to move on the floor during the kick. Once the kick makes contact with the target, it is immediately retracted at greater force than was used to push it out. The idea is that the kick will make contact and begin retracting before any force is pushed back into the kicker. Therefore, the kick does not require as solid a base of support as thrusting kicks.

Yoko Geri Kekomi

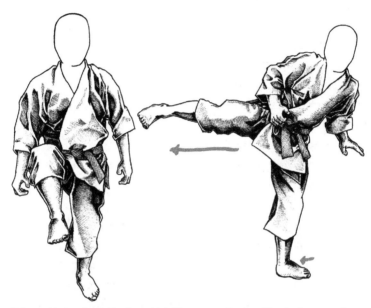

Yoko geri kekomi, or side thrust kick. The preparatory position is shown on the left, and the final kick position is shown on the right. The kick thrusts parallel to the floor toward the target. The body center is driven toward the target by the shift in the support leg; note the change in foot position through driving forward on the ball of the foot.

Yoko geri kekomi, or side thrust kick, is a very strong kick. It makes use of the inductor and gluteus muscles, and the hip is completely turned into the opponent at impact. The kick is executed by lifting the leg as if preparing for mae geri, but then the kicking leg lifts so that the shin is parallel to the floor and there is a direct line from the buttocks to the heel to the opponent. The leg then simply extends as if squatting, except that now the heel and blade of the foot are driving into the opponent. It is important to rotate the kicking foot downward as it extends to protect the hip joint of the kicking leg, and in particular the adductor muscles. While the kicking leg is extending, the support leg is also driving into the opponent. The heel of the supporting leg drives off the floor and rotates, so that the foot of the supporting leg is facing directly away from the opponent. This has the effect of allowing the hips to drive into the correct position and engage the buttocks and inductors of the supporting leg. Generally, when teaching this technique I break it down into six components rather than the traditional four: (1) first, lift the knee as if loading to mae geri. (2) Then lift the shin bone to the correct coiled position. The leg is effectively in the same tight load as for mae geri but angled so that it is flat to the floor, so that the hip, knee, and ankle are parallel to the floor, and the knee and ankle are pointing in a direct line to the target. The heel of the supporting leg should shift to the final position at this step. It is important to exhale here to allow the correct contraction of the abdominals. This allows better timing of the breath when steps 2 and 3 are combined later. (3) Naturally extend the leg. Putting some resistance on the leg (such as by using a workout band) or having someone hold onto the leg can help students understand the correct path of the leg. (4) Naturally retract the leg to position 2 (again, having some resistance can help teach this movement). (5) Bring the leg back to the chamber (position 1), rotating the support leg back to the original position as well, and (6) place the leg down. Once students understand this set of movements, I have them combine positions 2 and 3 as well as positions 4 and 5, connecting the breath, support heel, and kick impact into the same instant.

The body drive of this kick is quite substantial and originates from the drive of the supporting leg. As the kick is executed, the support leg is rotated on the ball of the foot, effectively driving the heel of the support leg along the floor toward the target. This in turn moves the body center toward the opponent and, if timed correctly, the body center will be in motion as the leg penetrates the target. In this way, additional body weight can be transferred to the target.

One important point is that yoko geri kekomi should very rarely be practiced with full power and speed unless a solid target is being hit. Driving the leg out in a straight line and stopping abruptly can cause joint separation. It is not good for students to do lots of repetitions of this kick at full power and speed in the air.

Fumikomi Geri and Fumikiri Geri

Fumikomi geri (stamping kick) and fumikiri geri (stamping cutting kick) are identical to yoko geri kekomi, with the exception of the target. In fumikomi geri, the target is the opponent's shin or instep, which are attacked by a downward stomping motion. Fumikiri geri, on the other hand, is driven into the knee joint. Even though both kicks are low, the position of the knee in the preparatory position should still remain high.

Yoko Tobi Geri

Yoko tobi geri, or flying side kick, is similar to yoko geri kekomi, except that the support leg is driven upward at the point of contact to a position similar to the preparatory position for yoko geri keage. It could be thought of as a tuck jump with one leg kicking out. It is important to synchronize the zenith of the jump with the tuck of the support leg, with the extension and impact of the kicking leg. A good way to practice this is to have a partner hold the extended kicking leg out while the person executing the kick jumps, pulling the support leg into the final position.

Roundhouse Kicks

The roundhouse (or turning) kick gets its name from its characteristic motion, which is horizontal to the floor. It is designed to kick around opponents and hit them from the side.

Mawashi Geri

Mawashi geri, the roundhouse kick, could be called a sideways front kick. The preparatory position has the kicking leg high and tight to the back (my pet name for this kick is "dog taking a pee kick" for this reason), the shin parallel to the floor, the foot dorsiflexed, and the femur in a straight line from the knee to the opposite hip. This position is maintained as the hips are rotated, and the supporting leg drives toward the opponent; this is achieved by rotating the supporting leg so that the foot is pointing away from the opponent, as in yoko geri kekomi. This has the effect of driving the body center toward the target. The kicking leg simultaneously extends toward the opponent as the body rotates in an arc. Ideally, impact is made at the same time as the heel of the supporting foot connects with the floor after its rotation. If done correctly, the shin bone of the kicking leg runs out on a smooth arc that is parallel to the floor, giving the illusion that the shin "telescopes" from the knee joint. The kicking weapon can be either the ball of the foot or the instep. To kick high, the hip must be opened wider in the load so that the femur is open and the whole femur and shank point to the target. It is not sufficient to simply point the knee toward the target. The shin in its arc must always remain equidistant from the floor.

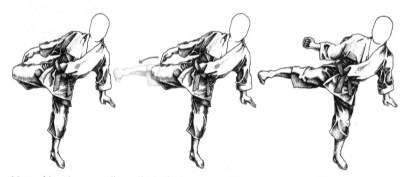

Mawashi geri, or roundhouse kick. The later part of the preparatory position is shown on the left, and the final kick position is shown on the right, with the transition in the middle. Note that the shank (shin bone) moves parallel to the floor as the kick is executed.

Ura Mawashi Geri

Ura mawashi geri, or hook kick, is the opposite of the roundhouse kick (mawashi geri) in that, rather than taking an outside-to-outside path, it takes an inside-to-outside path to the target. (Because it mirrors mawashi geri in this way, I include it in this section.) The simplest way to achieve this is to simply do a yoko geri kekomi kick and aim to the other side of the opponent's body. That is, if you are kicking with the right leg, kick to the left of your opponent so the heel is next to your opponent's face. Next, bend the knee and hit the opponent with the heel or sole of the foot while retracting the hips. As it is practiced more, the kick becomes much more fluid, but it is important not to make it too relaxed and "floppy," especially through the knee joint.

Back Kicks

Back kicks are the most powerful class of kicks in karate. They derive their power from the buttocks and using the heel as a striking surface.

Ushiro Geri

Ushiro geri, or back kick, is very similar to what a horse does when someone walks behind it. To execute the kick, the knee is lifted as in mae geri, and the leg then drives straight backward, brushing the knee of the support leg. At the point of contact, the back flexes, and the foot is pointing downward. The striking surface is the heel.

Conclusion

While there are many other variations of kicks—hooking, spinning, and jumping—it is important to practice the basic five kicks: mae geri, yoko geri keage, yoko geri kekomi, mawashi geri, and ushiro geri. If these kicks are practiced consistently, it becomes obvious that they supply the mechanics for all other kicks. Therefore, it could be argued that all other kicks simply derive from these basic five.

References

Bremaeker, M. D., and R. Faige. *Essential Book of Martial Arts Kicks*. Tokyo: Tuttle Publishing, 2010.

Kanazawa, H. *Black Belt Karate: The Intensive Course*. Tokyo: Kodansha International, 2006.

Nakayama, M. *Best Karate*. Vols. 5–6. New York: Kodansha USA, 1979.

Nakayama. M. *Dynamic Karate: Instruction by the Master*. Tokyo: Kodansha International, 1966.

Nishiyama, H., and R. C. Brown. *Karate: The Art of "Empty-Hand" Fighting*. Boston: Tuttle Publishing, 1960.

Okazaki, T., and M. V. Stricevic. *The Textbook of Modern Karate*. New York: Kodansha International, 1984.

Otsuka, H. *Wado Ryu Karate*. Hong Kong: Masters Publication, 1997.

Yamaguchi, G. *Goju Ryu Karate Do Kyohan*. Hamilton, ON: Masters Publication, 1999.

CHAPTER 8

Uchi: Striking Techniques

Uchi are a class of karate hand techniques that are often taken to be synonymous with striking. They are best described by their path of movement to the target relative to the long bone of the forearm (*1*). This means that in most cases the path is perpendicular to the forearm, and the striking surface is on one of the sides of the forearm or hand.

Principles of Uchi

Since the striking surface is often on the side of the limb, a variety of angles can be used to attack the target. In addition, the use of keage, kekomi, and ate (see chapter 18) can be employed across a variety of techniques, allowing many of the strikes to hit the target in multiple ways. In order to do this effectively, several universal principles need to be observed.

The first is the rotation of the radius and ulna. They need to be rotated sharply from a fully supinated to a fully pronated position, or from a fully pronated to a fully supinated position between the beginning and the end of the technique. This allows for the muscles of the forearm to tense at the same time as the hips and driving leg, using the breath to synchronize the tensing of these components. This also allows for the weapon to be completely formed at the point of contact.

The second is to understand what type of hip motion is being employed with which strike (see chapters 13 to 15). Snap (keage), thrust (kekomi), and smashing (ate) will have differing connections to the hip movement. In addition, as discussed in chapter 18, reinforcement of the body varies for each mode of hitting the target. While the individual movements will be discussed later, it is important to remember this point.

The third important point is to make sure that the correct weapon is used for the technique. It is vital that the weapon be tense and strong at the point of contact, otherwise the striking limb can be injured on impact.

Finally, understand how the final position of the strike connects to the torso and which muscles are engaged to hold the humerus and forearms in strong positions for the impact. Generally, these will be the same as in punching (tsuki) (chapter 6) and can be summarized as follows: only fully contract the chest (pectoralis) and back (latissimus dorsi) muscles at the point of impact. Contract them equally while letting the shoulders relax at the conclusion of the technique. Having a strong connection to the torso is important to get the body weight behind the strike.

Types of Strikes

Strikes can generally be divided into three categories: fist (kobushi), open (kaisho), and elbow (hiji). Fist strikes (kobushi uchi) hit the opponent with a closed hand, but not with seiken (the front two knuckles). Open strikes (kaisho uchi) are with an open hand but not with any weapons that are in the thrusting motion; striking surfaces are the surfaces of the hand that are not at the end of the long bone such as nukite. Hiji uchi, or elbow strikes, are powerful weapons and hit, of course, with the elbow.

The discussion of uchi is based from Okazaki Shihan's book *Textbook of Modern Karate*, as it has a superior listing of techniques compared to many other resource materials (*1–7*). However, where appropriate, I have included information from the others.

Fist Strikes (Kobushi Uchi)

The most common fist strikes (kobushi uchi) use uraken or tettsui (chapter 2) as weapons. Uraken refers to the backfist, and in particular the back of the front two knuckles. Of the uraken there are two types: otoshi uraken (downward backfist) and soto uraken (outward backfist). Tettsui refers to the bottom of the fist. Of the tettsui, there are four varieties: uchi kentsui (inward hammer), soto kentsui (outward hammer), otoshi kentsui (downward hammer), and kentsui hasami (double hammer).

Otoshi Uraken Uchi

Otoshi uraken, or downward backfist, is a smashing (ate) or thrusting (kekomi) striking technique. Quite often it moves in direct rotation with the hips; that is, the elbow moves in the same direction as the hip. It is initiated by moving the arm to an age uke, or rising block position; the elbow then drops sharply and directly downward to the same final position as in a cross block (soto ude uke—see next chapter); the elbow is about one fist width off the hip. In the process, the forearm is fully supinated to expose the backfist (uraken). The strong connection to the hip and strong forearm position (ninety degrees from the humerus) ensure that this technique is able to take full advantage of the body weight. In addition, the technique is normally in line with the base of support (rear leg) or is performed with a dropping motion to use gravity (e.g., Heian yondan movement #13 at the first kiai).

Soto Uraken Uchi

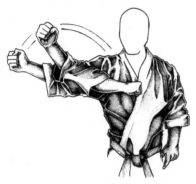

Soto uraken, or outward backfist, showing the semicircular path of the attacking limb.

Soto uraken, or outward backfist, is a keage, or snapping technique; therefore, it does not require a large base of support since it does not have to absorb much reaction force. The technique can be loaded in a lower block (gedan barai) type of load, where the arms cross in front of the body in a push-pull motion. The striking hand can be either above or below the covering (nonstriking) hand, depending on the application. The elbow pushes directly toward the target while the forearm is in a fully pronated position. Once the elbow is extended to its full position (pointing directly at the target), the elbow straightens, extending the forearm. The radius and ulna are supinated to expose uraken. The extension path should be soft and natural to the joint and on the angle comfortable for the practitioner. As soon as contact is made, the arm is snapped back to the bent elbow position and the forearm is pronated back. While the snapback is sharp, it is vital that it be relaxed and natural. If it is "muscled back," it will be more difficult to execute the follow-up technique. The hips snap and, depending on circumstance, can be forward or reverse rotation, but the body center always moves toward the opponent.

Interestingly, the technique can be changed a little for advanced practitioners by shifting from a natural fighting posture (kamae) using uraken to begin an attack. The hand that is out does not need to initially pull back to a preparatory position. In a real encounter this would be too slow. Rather, directly lift the elbow to point at the target while snapping the technique directly out and relaxing back. This integrated movement requires a thorough understanding of the basic movement described above.

Uchi Kentsui Uchi

Uchi kentsui, or inward hammerfist strike, is a strong ate or kekomi type of technique. Generally, it moves in a direct rotation with the hip and takes a path similar to the outside cross block (soto ude uke) (e.g., the shuto version is shown in the section "Uchi Shuto Uchi," below). The load is the same as in soto ude uke, with the humerus parallel to the ground. The wrist is fully pronated. The elbow swings downward on a direct diagonal motion accompanied by the hips moving to a half-facing position (hanmi), as if the elbow and hip were connected by a piece of string, while the wrist supinates to expose the hammerfist (tettsui). If the technique is completed on the gyaku side, the final position is shomen.

Soto Kentsui Uchi

Soto kentsui, or outward hammerfist strike, is also a strong smashing (ate) or thrusting (kekomi) technique. This loads the same way as soto uraken; however, tettsui is exposed rather than uraken, and the technique is not snapped back (the shuto version of this technique is shown below under "Soto Shuto Uchi"). Depending on distance and initial position, both direct rotation and translation movement of the hip can be employed. Distance to the target can also dictate how far the striking arm can extend. If the target were farther away, the practitioner would fully extend the elbow and use a forward stance with the hips half facing (zenkutsu dachi hanmi). If the opponent were close, the elbow would only be extended to a ninety-degree position and horse-riding stance (kiba dachi) would be used.

Otoshi Kentsui Uchi

Otoshi kentsui, or downward hammerfist strike, is almost identical to otoshi uraken, except that the hammerfist is exposed rather than the backfist.

Kentsui Hasami Uchi

Kentsui hasami, or double hammerfist strike, is a strong double-handed strike generally used to attack the floating ribs. To execute the technique, both hands are raised in a double rising block (age uke) position with the wrists fully pronated. Then the elbows are dropped sharply and directly to the sides, and the forearms are rotated to a fully supinated position. Since there is no hip rotation in this technique, it frequently uses other methods to derive power from the body center, including translation, elevation, and core connection. For this reason, it is often completed in a front-facing forward stance (zenkutsu dachi shomen).

Open-Handed Strikes (Kaisho Uchi)

Open-handed strikes include many kinds of strikes that do not use a closed fist. While there are many surfaces of the hand that can be used (see chapter 2), the focus here will be on shuto, haito, and teisho. Shuto refers to the blade edge of the hand between the wrist and the start of the little finger. Haito refers to the same region of the hand but on the thumb side. To make haito, it is important to tuck the thumb completely into the palm of the hand to expose the striking surface. Teisho refers to the palm heel of the hand and can refer either to the "meaty" part of the palm or the edge where the hand joins the wrist when the hand is extended upward.

Otoshi Shuto Uchi

Otoshi shuto uchi, or downward knife-hand strike, is the classic "karate chop." It is completed with much the same motion as otoshi kentsui uchi; however, the hand is open and the knife hand or shuto is the striking surface.

Uchi Shuto Uchi

Uchi shuto uchi, or inward knife-hand strike, often moves in direct rotation with the hips. The preparatory position is similar to soto ude uke, except that the hand is in a shuto position with the wrist fully pronated. Since the head or neck is often the target, the elbow moves in a direct line to the target and the arm extends as the wrist sharply supinates. The hand hits the target at a thirty- to forty-five-degree vector, driving the target both back and on the angle.

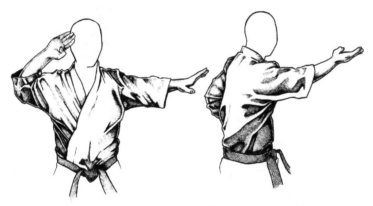

Uchi shuto uchi, or inward knife-hand strike. The preparatory position is shown on the left, and the final position is shown on the right.

Soto Shuto Uchi

Soto shuto uchi, or outward knife-hand strike, often moves in a reverse rotation or vibration with the hips. (For the concept of hip vibration, see chapter 14). The beginning position of the hand is similar to knife-hand block (shuto uke), with the striking hand across the body, palm facing the ear. The elbow then drives toward the target, and the arm extends, pronating the wrist to expose the striking surface (shuto). For this strike, the opposite hand does not need to be used as a covering hand in the normal push-pull motion. Generally, if practitioners have the luxury of using a full rotation from front face (shomen) to half face (hanmi), they will use a full covered load. If they are already in hanmi, they will just use core connection to execute the strike and not make use of a covering hand.

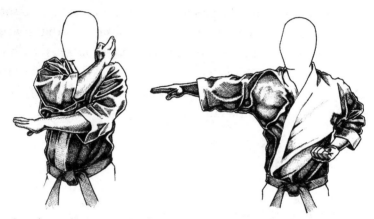

Soto shuto uchi, or outward knife-hand strike. The preparatory position is shown on the left, and the final position is shown on the right.

Uchi Haito Uchi

Uchi haito uchi, or inward ridge-hand strike, is performed from the normal beginning position of choku zuki (straight punch), with the fist in a fully supinated position and the hip in half face (hanmi). The hip then rotates to full face (shomen), and the hand is released from the hip and extends naturally in an arcing angle with the hip. Meanwhile, the wrist rotates to a fully pronated position with the palm down, exposing the ridge hand, which makes contact with the target—usually the temple or the neck—at a ninety-degree angle.

Soto Haito Uchi

Soto haito uchi, or outward ridge-hand strike, is similar to uchi haito uchi, except the hand rotates from a pronated position in the load to a supinated position for the strike.

Age Teisho Uchi

Age teisho uchi, or rising palm-heel strike, is almost more of a thrust than a strike since the attacking surface is in line with the forearm. The technique is almost identical to a straight punch to the face (choku zuki jodan), except that the hand is flexed and the fingers are tucked to form the palm heel (teisho) weapon. The target for this attack is anything prominent, such as the underside of the jaw or the nose.

Uchi Teisho Uchi

Uchi teisho uchi, or inward palm-heel strike, rotates with the hips. This technique begins in the choku zuki position described above for uchi haito uchi. As the hip rotates to full face (shomen), the hand is released from the hip, and the arm arcs with the hip as it extends. The wrist remains almost in a relaxed flexion. At the point of contact, which is triggered by the hip connection, the wrist extends and tenses as the hand forms teisho.

Elbow Strikes (Hiji Uchi)

Elbow strikes are a very strong weapon in karate, primarily due to their increased connection to the body through a short lever. In addition, the elbow is a hard weapon that can be used to hit a target with a lot of force. One important point, however, is to make sure the wrist is in the correct position (fully pronated) when the elbow strikes. This wrist position tightens the tendons in the forearm and elbow, and makes the weapon less prone to damage.

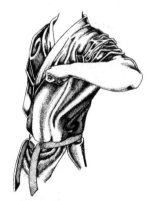

Side elbow thrust, or yoko empi uchi.

The major differentiating factor in hiji (empi or elbow strike) uchi is the direction or vector along which the elbow travels. We will discuss five different types of elbow (empi) strikes: mae (front), yoko (side), tate (rising), otoshi (downward), and yoko mawashi (side round).

Interestingly, some hiji uchi do not hit the target perpendicular to the forearm, which is required for strikes. But each hiji technique begins in a way that is similar to its corresponding strike (through an arc). This is true even though in some cases (yoko, mae otoshi) the hiji technique makes contact parallel to the forearm. For this reason, all hiji or empi techniques fall under uchi.

Mae Empi Uchi

Mae empi uchi, or front elbow strike, is interesting in that the final weapon forms well in advance of the actual strike, and it is the body's translation into the target that delivers the impact. This type of technique is a true smashing technique (ate waza), literally smashing through the target.

The technique begins in the normal front punch (choku zuki) position chambered on the hip. While stepping forward into a half-facing forward stance (zenkutsu dachi hanmi), the hand is rotated so that it sits palm down in a fist on the breastbone, with the elbow pointing directly forward. Ideally this shape is formed well before contact with the target. The rear leg then can drive the elbow directly into the target. Note that the arm does not need to move once in position; it just needs to be held in the preformed position for this technique to be effective.

Yoko Empi Uchi

Yoko empi uchi, or side elbow strike, is performed from kiba dachi. It is executed in a manner similar to soto uraken uchi, except that the arm does not extend to expose the backfist. Rather, the wrist pronates so that it first stops directly over the nipple closest to the target—see the illustration above in the section "Elbow Strikes

(Hiji Uchi)." This biological landmark is extremely useful for aligning the elbow in the front-to-back planes and ensuring correct alignment of the elbow to the body. In addition, it is vital to connect the horse-riding stance (kiba dachi) properly at the point of impact. This allows the drive of the elbow forward to couple with the translational motion of the hips connecting to a solid base at impact.

Tate (Age) Empi Uchi

Tate (age) empi uchi, or rising elbow strike, is completed with a direct rotation of the hips. It begins in a choku zuki preparatory position on the hip. The elbow drives forward and upward while the hand rotates—still tightly connected to the humerus—from a supinated to the pronated position by the ear, with the palm adjacent to the ear. Care must be taken not to punch oneself at the conclusion of the technique.

As the technique is executed, it is important to keep the elbow fully flexed and not to allow it to extend. Keep the hand close to the shoulder throughout. Exceptions to this rule can include striking the opponent with the fist as the technique extends. For example, one could use ura or tate zuki, then in the same motion transition to tate empi uchi.

Otoshi Empi Uchi

Otoshi empi uchi, or downward elbow strike, is identical to otoshi uraken uchi, with the exception that the wrist remains fully pronated at the point of contact.

Yoko Mawashi Empi Uchi

Yoko mawashi empi uchi, or round side elbow strike, begins in a choku zuki preparatory position on the hip. It is executed in a direct rotation with the hip from a half-face (hanmi) to a full-face (shomen) position. As the hip rotates, the fist pronates as the elbow arcs round, so that the fist ends on the breastbone if the technique is executed in half-face forward stance (zenkutsu dachi hanmi).

Conclusion

While there are many other strike variations using different weapons (for example, haishu uchi), it is important to note that generally they can come from one of four angles: to either side, up, or down. This means that, depending on the weapon, they can be executed using an uchi, soto, age, or otoshi preparatory position and execution. In addition, it is important to remember that the final rotation of the wrist and movement of the hips help time the technique and connect it to the body.

Notes

1. E. Schmeisser, *Advanced Karate-Do* (St. Louis: Focus Publications, 1994).
2. G. Funakoshi, *Karate Do Kyohan: Master Text for the Way of the Empty Hand* (San Diego: Neptune Publications, 2005).
3. H. Kanazawa, *Black Belt Karate: The intensive Course* (Tokyo: Kodansha International, 2006).
4. M. Nakayama, *Dynamic Karate: Instruction by the Master* (Tokyo: Kodansha International, 1966), 308.
5. H. Nishiyama and R. C. Brown, *Karate: The Art of "Empty-Hand" Fighting* (Boston: Tuttle Publishing, 1960).
6. T. Okazaki and M. V. Stricevic, *The Textbook of Modern Karate* (New York: Kodansha International, 1984).
7. R. L. Rielly, *Secrets of Shotokan Karate* (Boston: Tuttle Publishing, 2000), x, 246.

CHAPTER 9

Uke: Blocking Techniques

Introduction to Uke

The word uke is derived from ukeru, which literally means "to receive" but can also mean "catch," "undergo," "be exposed to," "preparedness," "stop or parry a blow," "block," or "sustain a hit" (gojublogger.com). This class of techniques, along with dachi (stance), uchi (strike), tsuki (thrust), and keri (kick), together make up the total arsenal of fundamental karate-do techniques. Generally, uke requires that the hip move the body in a rotational fashion, often to the hanmi, or half-face position, along with a cross-body elbow movement. Oftentimes these movements allow the practitioner to parry or block an attack, but they can also have a wider spectrum of applications and can be used as strikes, locks, or thrusts to incapacitate an opponent. This is why "to receive" seems far more accurate as a translation for uke compared to the usual translation, "block," that is prevalent in most dojo.

This chapter focuses on the basic uke of karate-do. We will discuss how these movements can have multiple applications for a single movement and how the movements can be applied in multiple ways. This serves as an example for all karate techniques.

The Five Basic Uke of Karate and Their Mechanics

When beginners start in Shotokan karate, they are taught five basic uke. These are lower block (gedan barai), rising block (age uke), outside cross block (soto ude uke), inside cross block (uchi ude uke), and knife hand (shuto uke).

Gedan Barai

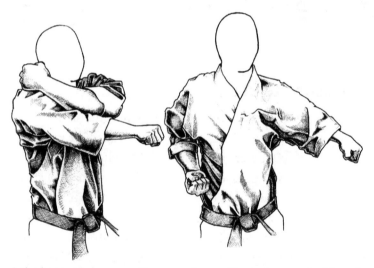

Gedan barai, or lower sweep. The preparatory position is shown on the left, and the final position is shown on the right.

Gedan barai literally means "lower sweep," and it refers to the movement of the elbow and arm moving in a diagonal direction from shoulder to hip, crossing the body in the process. The final position has the blocking arm straight and the elbow one fist width from the closest hip, while opposite hand sits on the hip. The motion of the block draws the blocking hand across the body from where it is initially placed at the opposite ear, and the other hand is pushed straight out in front. The block is executed by sweeping the elbow across the body as the opposite hand is pulled back in a roughly diagonal sweeping motion. To complete the movement of the block, the radius and ulna bones of the blocking forearm must be rotated away from the body to connect the technique. When executed from an initial front hip facing position, the hip moves in the opposite direction to that of the block. This is reversed when the block initiates in a half-facing position and the body rotates in the same direction as the block.

Age Uke

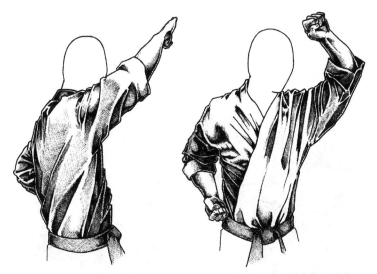

Age uke, or rising block. The preparatory position is shown on the left, and the final position is shown on the right.

Age uke means "rising block," and refers to the motion of the block moving in a rising fashion. It is loaded by putting the covering hand in the final position of the block, with the hand open in a shuto (open-handed) position (see below), while the opposite fist is sitting on the hip. Age uke is executed by driving the hand on the hip, following the rotational motion of the hip, like an uppercut, keeping the elbow close to the body. The hand that had been the raised blocking hand in the initial position now moves back to the hip (the covering hand) in time with the blocking hand. It is important to not drop this hand too early, as it can be used to keep the head covered throughout the motion. Once the blocking hand is level with the chin, the radius and ulna are rotated away from the body, which rotates the forearm from a vertical position relative to the floor to a forty-five-degree position. The elbow moves in a straight, vertical line in the same direction as the hip movement. The final position for the elbow is the same as kizami zuki. The fist position of the final block is a fist and a thumb's length from the forehead, and the wrist is in line with the nose.

Soto Ude Uke

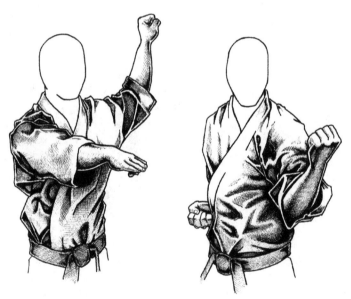

Soto ude uke, or cross block from the outside, moving inward. The preparatory position is shown on the left, and the final position is shown on the right.

Soto ude uke means "cross block from the outside, moving inward." Like age uke, the elbow in soto ude uke moves in the same direction as the hip. The preparatory position for the block has the covering arm straight out in front, while the humerus of the blocking arm is held parallel to the floor to the side. The forearm is fully rotated so that the fist is facing away from the body and can be held either at right angles or tucked close to the ear. The block is executed by rotating the hip to half face (hanmi). The blocking hand is dragged downward with the hip as the covering hand is drawn back to the hip. The blocking elbow is drawn downward. By combining the hip movement with the dropping of the elbow, the block moves in a diagonal direction across the body. The arm does not shift laterally in the shoulder joint during the movement. The downward motion of the blocking hand rotates the radius and ulna toward the body center, connecting the hand to the body. The final position for the block has the draw hand (the hand pulling back to the body) on the hip, with the blocking elbow one fist width from the hip and the forearm at ninety degrees to the humerus. The forearm and fist are fully rotated toward the body, and the arm is somewhat perpendicular to the floor, with the gap between the middle and ring finger in line with the nose.

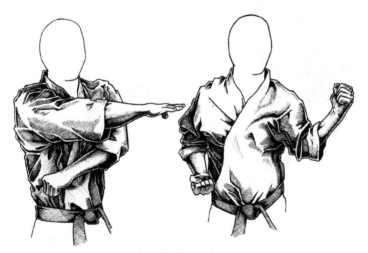

Uchi ude uke, or cross block from inside, moving outside. The preparatory position is shown on the left, and the final position is shown on the right.

Uchi Ude Uke

Uchi ude uke means "cross block from inside moving outside." The preparatory position has the covering hand straight out in front of the body, while the blocking hand sits across the body near the hip, palm down. The block is executed by pulling the covering hand back to the hip, simultaneously moving the opposite elbow horizontally across the body while the hip moves in the opposite direction. The forearm is rotated quickly so that the fist faces inward while it is simultaneously pushed outward and away from the body. In the final position, the elbow is one fist width off the hip, and the forearm is ninety degrees from the humerus, facing inward, where the gap between the middle and ring finger is in line with the nose. The blocking hand always moves to the outside of the retracting covering hand.

Shuto Uke

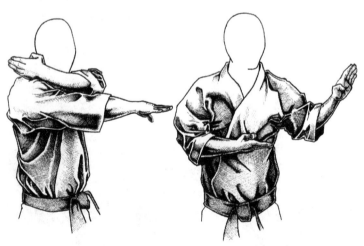

Shuto uke, or knife-hand block. The preparatory position is shown on the left, and the final position is shown on the right.

Shuto uke is very similar dynamically to gedan barai, with the exception of the final position. The preparatory position is the same. It is dynamically similar to gedan barai as well, with the exception of the final position. In the final position, the covering hand is not drawn completely back to the hip but rather to the midline of the body, just below the xiphoid process in the shuto position (palm up). The blocking hand rotates the forearm completely away from the body (palm away), and the elbow finishes one fist's distance from the body, the forearm at ninety degrees from the humerus and the hand in the shuto position. Normally, the hips move in the opposite direction to the hip.

The table at the end of this chapter shows that most of these blocks have several points in common. First, the blocking elbow moves from one side of the body to the other in the movement—up and down, side to side, or diagonally. Second, the covering hand is always out in front of the body in the preparatory position. Third, the hips move with the block when the blocking hand is loaded to the outside of the body; it does not cross the midline. The hips move opposite to the block when the blocking hand travels across the body—in other words, when the hand needs to cross the midline. Finally, the final position of the elbow is one fist width off the front hanmi hip (with the exception of age uke).

The Principle of the Five Uke and Their Relation to Other More "Advanced" Blocks

The final position of many of the five blocks can be executed at different levels. For example, uchi ude uke can be executed at two levels in addition to the normal chudan, or stomach, level (elbow one fist width from the hip). Jodan uchi ude uke, or upper inside cross block, is executed at a final position where the humerus is shoulder height, with the forearm at right angles and the fist pointing outward from the body. Gedan uchi ude uke, or lower inside cross block, is performed the same way as regular uchi ude uke, except the final position of the blocking arm is one fist width from the hip and the forearm has a slight curve at the elbow as compared to the standard ninety-degree bend. It is rotated outward. This illustrates that the principle behind the block can be maintained irrespective of technique. Each of the five basic blocks can be analyzed similarly.

Based on the idea that the principle of the movement is almost more important than the technique itself, it is apparent that often more-advanced blocks—those introduced later on in karate training—are simply derived from the five basic blocks. Some simple examples include morote uke, or augmented block, which is simply an augmented uchi uke using the draw hand for support on the blocking hand. Juji uke, or x-block, is simply a gedan barai coupled with gyaku zuki. Jodan haiwan uke, ude soete (the block from the first movement from Heian nidan) is a combination of jodan uchi ude uke and age uke.

Application of Five Basic Blocks Using Gedan Barai as an Example

By the nature and complexity of their movement, blocks can represent an opportunity to receive the opponent, no matter what attack was delivered, and counter with a variety of movements. The block in itself may therefore represent a very comprehensive method for self-defense. For example, consider gedan barai. The technique has two major parts: the preparatory position and the execution. These parts consist of both arms moving in different (often opposing) directions in a contracting (load) and expanding (execution) movement. By employing every part of the movement at a number of ranges, it is possible to apply the principles behind these techniques in many ways.

The complete gedan barai movement consists of multiple parts, each of which can have a separate meaning. This is especially true in relation to an opponent. Each part of the technique can be associated with blocking an attack directed at a different target.

In addition, the block can also become a strike, a joint lock, or a throw.

Gedan barai begins with the hips square to the front, with one hand across the body and the fist by the ear. The opposite hand is straight out in front and can be in the lower- or middle-level straight punch or gedan or chudan choku zuki position. Both hands and movement can be analyzed. The hand moving to the ear can be used as a tsuki on the way by taking a straight path out to an opponent's midsection. The movement to the ear can also be used as a sweeping block (nagashi uke), with either the flat of the hand or the fist striking the opponent's attacking weapon. The opposite hand thrust can be a reverse punch (gyaku zuki), a punching block (zuki uke), or a reverse lower block (gyaku gedan barai). In the execution of gedan barai, the blocking hand sweeps down the extended arm as it pulls back to the hip. This movement can either be gedan barai or a hammerfist strike (tettsui uchi). Therefore, it is possible to strike an opponent three times with this block. For example, if an attacker went to punch a defender in the face, the defender could attack when the opponent attacks (sen no sen timing) and hit the attacker as the punch is initiated by striking directly to the abdomen. Then the punch to the face could be blocked with nagashi uke. Simultaneously, the defender can hit with the opposite hand using choku zuki, and then the loaded (nagashi uke) hand could strike down with tettsui uchi. Gedan barai also allows defenders to completely cover their body at the jodan, chudan, and gedan levels using gyaku gedan barai (chudan), nagashi uke (jodan), and gedan barai (gedan). No matter where the defender is attacked, there is a possible defense.

In addition to these classical strike/block/punch defenses, if the target area is brought closer, the techniques of gedan barai can be used as a joint lock or to break a grip. Either hand can be grabbed, and gedan barai can be used to strike the hand using the gedan barai itself. Alternatively, the movement of the blocking hand being

The Five Basic Uke of Shotokan Karate: Important Points

Block	Blocking hand preparatory position	Covering hand preparatory position	Hip movement relative to elbow	Final covering hand position	Final blocking position of elbow	Final forearm position
Gedan barai	By opposite ear, palm facing ear	Straight out in front	Opposite direction to elbow from shoulder to hip	Hip	Hip in hanmi, elbow one fist width off	Straight with rest of arm, radius and ulna rotated away from body
Age uke	Blocking arm side hip	In final blocking position, but open hand	Vertical with elbow from hip to kizami zuki	Hip	Hip in hanmi, elbow in kizami zuki position	Bent at 90 degrees relative to humerus, 45 degrees to floor, radius and ulna rotated away from body
Soto ude uke	In line with shoulder, parallel to ground, wrist rotated away from body	Straight out in front	Diagonal downward with hip	Hip	Hip in hanmi, elbow one fist width off	Vertical to floor, bent at 90 degrees relative to humerus, wrist rotated toward body
Uchi ude uke	On opposite hip, palm down	Straight out in front	Horizontally in opposite direction to hip	Hip	Hip in hanmi, elbow one fist width off	Vertical to floor, bent at 90 degrees relative to humerus, wrist rotated toward body
Shuto uke	By opposite ear, palm facing ear	Straight out in front	Opposite direction to elbow from shoulder to hip	Midline of body, just below xiphoid process	Hip in hanmi, elbow one fist width off	Vertical to floor, bent at 90 degrees relative to humerus, wrist rotated away from body, hand in shuto

brought up to the ear is sufficient to break the grip. In addition, if the defender uses the gyaku gedan barai as a block and then traps the attacker's hand, the defender may strike the elbow joint (on either side) of the opponent's arm to move him into a more compliant posture. It is also important to point out the hikite, or pulling movement, of the draw hand returning to the hip, especially after trapping an attacker's hand. The hand rolls inward as it pulls back to the hip, also rotating the opponent's arm and presenting additional targets along the arm, or positioning the body in such a way that the attacker is unbalanced.

If the range is brought closer, so that the defender is standing hip to hip with the opponent, then the gedan barai may be used as a reaping throw (see chapter 10) over the defender's front leg. Or, alternatively, if the opponent grabs the defender from behind, the load hand (up by the ear) may be used to grab the opponent and the block may be executed as a hip throw.

Can These Concepts Be Carried Further?

This different way of thinking about blocks can also be carried over to virtually any karate technique, including thrusts, strikes, and kicks. This demonstrates that karate, while outwardly simple, is very complex. There are many ways its techniques can be applied, depending on distance, angle, and relative body position. Additionally, it is important to remember that every part of the movement can be used to some degree in defending oneself. This includes all transitional movements for both the attacking and the draw hand, as well as any leg and hip movement. The variety is only limited by the practitioner's imagination.

References

INTERNET

http://gojublogger.files.wordpress.com/2012/03/uke1.jpg

BOOKS

Funakoshi, G. *Karate-Dō Kyōhan: The Master Text.* Tokyo: Kodansha International, 1973.

Nakayama, M. *Best Karate.* Tokyo: Kodansha International, 1977.

Nakayama, M. *Dynamic Karate: Instruction by the Master.* Tokyo: Kodansha International, 1966.

Okazaki, T., and M. V. Stricevic. *The Textbook of Modern Karate.* Tokyo: Kodansha International, 1984.

CHAPTER 10

Kuzushi: Techniques of Breaking Balance

To break an opponent's balance (kuzushi), his center of gravity needs to be moved out of the base of support. In karate there are many techniques that can be used to do this. In chapter 12, we will discuss the theory of center of gravity and how balance is maintained and broken. While techniques for breaking balance abound in karate, they are not always stressed and must be drawn out of the techniques that have multiple applications. So let us briefly look at some techniques drawn from arts that make heavy use of breaking balance. In particular, we will discuss some of the specialized techniques in judo and aikido and then translate these principles back to Shotokan karate.

Types of Techniques That Break Balance

Before discussing balance-breaking techniques useful in karate, it is worthwhile to think about judo and aikido. Mikami Takayuki sensei once pointed out to me that the difference between karate and judo was simply in the fighting strategy. In karate we hit, then take the opponent to the floor, whereas in judo the opponent is first taken to the floor, then hit.

Judo

The judo curriculum has major parts: nagae-waza (throws), katame-waza (immobilizing, strangling, dislocation, or key holds), and ate-waza (blocks and strikes). Of the three, nagae-waza is the most important for our discussion about breaking balance. Nagae-waza is broken down into tachi-waza (standing throws) and sutemi-waza (throws from the ground). Tachi-waza includes ashi-waza (foot or leg throws), koshi-waza (hip throws), and te-waza. There are two kinds of te-waza: shoulder throws and hand-and-arm throws. Throws from the ground (sutemi-waza) come in two varieties as well: ma-sutemi-waza (throwing with one's back on the ground) and yoko-sutemi-waza (throwing with one's side on the ground) (*1, 2*).

In addition, judo has kata based on these throws. The one of particular interest for this discussion is the nagae-no kata, which contains fifteen basic throws[3] (three throws from each of the five categories) (*1, 2*). They are as follows:

Te-waza (arm throws)	Uki-otoshi (floating drop)
	Kata-seoki (shoulder throw)
	Kata-guruma (shoulder wheel)
Koshi-waza (hip throws)	Uki-goshi (floating loin)
	Hara-goshi (sweeping loin)
	Tsuri-komi-goshi (lift pull loin)

3. For an excellent reference for each of the throws listed here (with pictures and explanations), I suggest reading either Klinger-Klingerstorff (1953) or Otaki and Drager (1983)—see references at the end of this chapter.

Ashi-waza (foot and leg throws)	Okuri-ashi-barai (sweeping ankle throw)
	Sasae-tsuri-komi-ashi (propping, drawing, ankle throw)
	Uchi-mata (inner thigh)
Ma-sutemi-waza (falling or sacrifice throw with one's back on the ground)	Tomoe-nage (stomach throw)
	Ura-nage (rear throw)
	Sumi-gaeshi (corner throw)
Yoko-sutemi-waza (throws effected with one's side on the ground)	Yoko-game (side body drop)
	Yoko-guruma (side wheel)
	Uki-waza (floating throw)

The key point in this discussion is that by looking at the curriculum of judo, we can start to identify key principles for breaking balance that are applicable to karate. In judo, the two fundamental points are: (1) be able to pull opponents' center of gravity outside of their base. It is best not to use strength on strength but rather to have an understanding of the strong and weak points of their stance and exploit it. (2) Understand the fulcrums of both your own and your opponents' body that allow you to manipulate them to a correct throwing position. In judo, these fulcrums are the feet, ankles, knees, hips, shoulders, and head.

Aikido

Broadly speaking, aikido has two types of techniques: immobilizations and projections (3). In basic aikido, there are seven immobilizations (ikkyo, nikyo, sankyo, yonkyo, gokyo, shoho nagae, and kote gaeshi) and many projections (twenty-eight are listed in reference 3). An immobilization is defined as the defender maintaining contact with the aggressor throughout the immobilization. A projection is defined as the defender losing contact with the aggressor after the technique is applied. Immobilizations and projections can be used in combination to allow for defenses against many forms of attack.[4]

Aikido relies upon both of the key points mentioned above for judo. For point 1, moving opponents' center of gravity beyond their base, this is done through a refined dynamic sphere of movement that moves the opponent through their weak point or in the direction they are moving, in a circular fashion. For point 2, understanding fulcrums, aikido makes keen use of the wrist, elbow, shoulder, hip, knee, ankle, and neck.

Karate Throws

In *Karate-Do Kyohan*, Funakoshi Gichin mentions throwing techniques (*4*). He names nine techniques in particular. (The names of the techniques vary depending on the translation of *Karate-Do Kyohan*. For this book we are using the 2005 translation by Suzuki-Johnson and not the translation by Oshima sensei.) The first is called byo-bu daoshi (folding screen topple). In judo this technique is similar to o-soto-gari (major exterior reaping). The second is koma-nage (spinning top throw). In aikido this motion is similar to ikkyo. The third is kubi-wa (neck ring), which is similar in principle to many of the aikido neck manipulations. The fourth is kata-sha-rin (shoulder wheel), which is similar to o-soto-guruma (major outer wheel). The fifth is tsubame-gaeshi (swallow return), which is similar to the yama-arashi (mountain storm) of judo. The sixth is yari-dama (spearing throw), which looks similar to kata-sha-rin but expands the opponent's extended arm rather than using the opponent's neck as a fulcrum. It is similar to the judo technique kata-guruma (shoulder wheel). The seventh is called tani-otoshi (gorge drop); this is almost identical to uki-goshi (floating loin) used in judo. The eighth is ude-wa (arm ring), which seems not to have an

---

4. For an excellent description of many of the principles and techniques described in this section, see Westbrook and Ratti (1970)—see references at the end of this chapter.

equivalent in judo or aikido but is very similar to the "shoot" used in shoot fighting in Brazilian jujitsu. The ninth is gyaku-zuchi (upside-down hammer), similar to the judo kata-guruma (shoulder wheel).[5]

While Funakoshi formally describes these techniques, it is easy to see that they are simply applications of basic Shotokan karate techniques. For example, the table below shows the approximate correspondence among techniques from Funakoshi, judo and aikido, and Shotokan. This indicates the strong conservation of movement across Shotokan techniques that can be applied differently depending on the distance or body position the technique can be applied at. As one studies the kata, possibilities for throws and locks become more apparent in the rotations, blocks, punches, strikes, and kicks.

Funakoshi Throws and Proposed Equivalents

Funakoshi Technique	Proposed Equal Judo/ Aikido Technique	Kihon Shotokan Estimate
Byo-bu daoshi	O-soto-gari	Oi zuki
Koma-nage	Ikkyo	Soto ude uke
Kubi-wa	Aikido neck projections	Mawashi zuki
Kata-sha-rin	O-soto-guruma	Manji uke
Tsubame-gaeshi	Yama-arashi	Juji uke (applied in reverse position)
Yari-dama	Kata-guruma	Gedan barai
Tani-otoshi	Uki-goshi	Gyaku zuki performed during mawate
Ude-wa	"Shoot" in Brazilian jiu-jitsu	Gedan barai during mawate
Gyaku-zuchi	Kata-guruma	Uchi uke

---

5. All of these throws are described fully in Funakoshi's *Karate-do Kyohan* (2005), translation by Suzuki-Johnson.

Foot Sweeps

One other important set of balance-breaking techniques some-what represented in judo but much more refined in karate are the ashi barai, or foot sweeps (5). These techniques are based on unbalancing opponents by directly interfering with their base. This is achieved by sweeping the foot along a weak line of technique. This is generally the line where balance is the weakest; for example, when the opponent is stepping forward, the weak line of technique is in the direction from heel to toe. Therefore, a sweep along this direction pushing the heel away from the opponent will result in unbalancing. The distribution of the opponent's weight is also important to consider, especially if the opponent is stationary or in transition. This can be achieved either by attacking the foot with less weight on it if the opponent is stationary (back leg of zenkutsu dachi) or, alternatively, attacking as the weight is transitioning onto the weight-bearing leg (e.g., just before the front foot of zen-kutsu dachi is being placed). There are two major types of sweep: to the front or rear leg (the front leg sweep is pictured below) and to both legs (5).

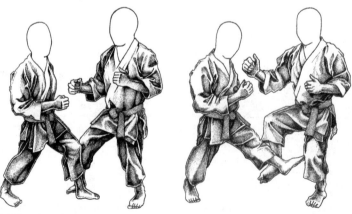

Ashi barai, or foot sweep.

Sweeps are very effective tools for a number of reasons. In the best-case scenario, the opponent will lose balance and fall to the ground. In a worst-case scenario, the opponent will feel the sweep attempt on their foot and momentarily lose concentration, allowing for an opening. In many cases, the normal effect is somewhere in between, where the opponent loses some balance but is able to recover. However, during that time opponents are focused on their balance and not on the person in front of them, leaving them open to attack.

As briefly discussed above, normally the foot is swept in the direction that expands the limb away from the body center (often the way it is pointing; for example, the opponent's front foot of zenkutsu dachi should be shifted from heel to toe direction, and not to the side). This direction is easier to move and expands the opponent's base in an unexpected direction. If swept toward the body center (to the side or too high), the technique could be ineffective—or, in a training situation, *too* effective, leading to injury to your partner's knee or ankle.

Mental Balance

The concept of foot sweeps brings up one other important point. Balance is a biological priority. We humans have adapted to standing upright, so if our balance is threatened, our recovery can take precedent, often to the detriment of the task at hand. While this topic is discussed in chapter 11, here let it be said that the value of techniques that leverage this reflex cannot be overstated.

It is important to work with students to make them more comfortable with losing balance. Careful instruction about what to do when in an unbalanced situation can lead to better control of their mental focus and less disruption overall. In this connection, practice in breaking falls (ukemi), as well as actually being thrown or swept, can be beneficial.

Important Principles (What Have We Learned?)

By investigating aikido and judo, we have learned several major concepts important in breaking physical balance (kuzushi).

The first is to move opponents' center of gravity outside their base, creating an unstable equilibrium. In judo, this is done by creating a tsuri-komi (or lift pull), while in aikido it is through the use of the dynamic sphere. The key is not to use force on force, where stronger opponents will win, but rather to move them in the direction they are already moving or in a direction where they are weak or not reinforced. In addition, the entire body, especially the body center, must be used for this purpose.

The second major point is that both judo and aikido use the main joints as leverage. These include the neck, shoulder, elbow, wrist, hip, knee, and ankle. With respect to the head, hip, and knee, a simple movement can go a long way toward shifting the opponent's center of gravity. An additional point is that, in general, it is better to be in a more stable position than the opponent (e.g., in the case of the hip throw, the thrower's hips should be lower than the opponent's).

Through our study of karate, especially kata, we can easily see that karate is rife with throwing and unbalancing applications. With simple techniques, depending on distance and body position relative to the opponent, throwing applications can be applied with ease.

Finally, it can be seen that techniques for breaking balance are important, especially since any modification to opponents' stability can override their attention to the task at hand. This can break their mental balance and allow the practitioner to decisively take the advantage.

Notes

1. H. Klinger-Klingerstorff, *Judo & Judo-Do* (London: H. Jenkins, 1953), 144.
2. T. Otaki and D. F. Draeger, *Judo: Formal Techniques* (Tokyo: Tuttle Publishing, 1983).
3. A. Westbrook and O. Ratti, *Aikido and the Dynamic Sphere* (Hong Kong: Tuttle Publishing Co., 1970).
4. G. Funakoshi, *Karate Do Kyohan: Master Text for the Way of the Empty Hand* (San Diego: Neptune Publications, 2005).
5. M. Nakayama, *Best Karate* (Tokyo: Kodansha International, 1977).

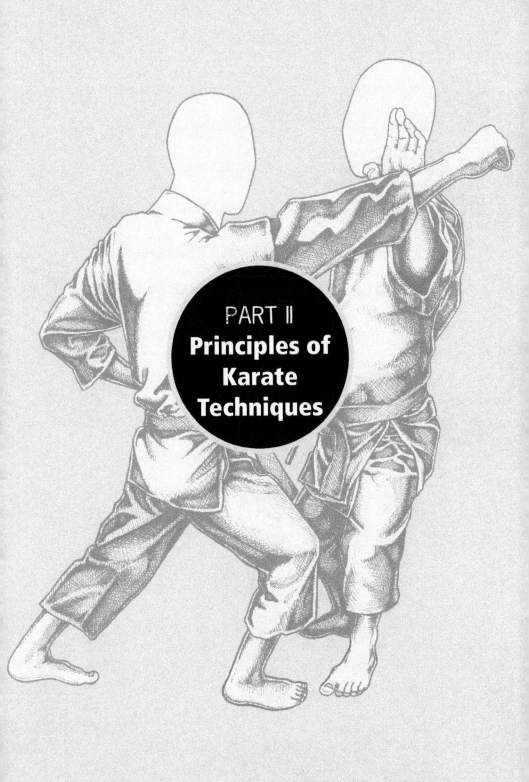

PART II
**Principles of
Karate
Techniques**

CHAPTER 11

How the Body Works: Joints and Muscles

The skeletal muscles and joints of the body exist to provide an articulation system for the skeleton and are a means of locomotion for the body. In the mammalian body plan, muscles are arranged in agonist-antagonist fashion. This can be likened to two opposing springs. They are set up this way because muscles can only contract or shorten. The mechanisms by which muscles contract will not be discussed here, but the sliding filament hypothesis is a wonderful story involving interesting players, including myosin, actin, calcium, endoplasmic reticulum, ATP, and many other biological terms. The major point is that in order for a limb to extend, it requires the shortening of one muscle, the agonist, and the relaxation of the opposing muscle, the antagonist. For the same limb to retract, the roles of the muscles reverse.

The body has several major skeletal muscle configurations. Each type allows for slightly different movement. The first configuration is circular; these muscles surround openings of sphincters. The second types are convergent, the muscle fibers converging to a single spot where they connect to the bone to maximize the force of muscle contraction (the trade-off is that they do not contract over a long distance). The third type is parallel. In this case, the fibers are lined up parallel to the bone and joint they are articulating. This gives them a long distance for contraction, but they are not very strong. The forth type is pennate, of which there are three types: unipennate, bipennate, and multipennate. Since they are arranged at an angle, somewhere between ten to eighty degrees relative to the bone and joint they are articulating, they produce very short but strong contractions. The fifth are fusiform, which are muscles that are parallel and slightly wider at their centers; this wider center allows for stronger contractions.

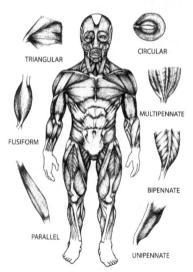

Major muscle configurations of the body.

Muscles connect to the skeleton via tendons at key points that allow for articulation or movement. The human skeleton is made up of 206 bones, and ligaments connect these bones to each other. The point at which each bone is connected is called a joint. There are several types of joints in the human body, each allowing for different kinds of articulation. The first type is called a pivot joint. This allows rotational movement, such as the rotation of the radius and ulna at the wrist (allowing for wrist rotation). The second type is a hinge joint, which allows for flexion and extension along a single axis, such as elbows and knees. The third type of joint is the ball-and-socket joint, which allows movement along three axes: flexion and extension, rotation, and adduction (drawing near the trunk) and abduction (drawing away from the trunk).

Examples of these joints are the hips and shoulders.

How these can relate to karate movements, in particular to hand techniques, is important to understand. First, we will discuss how the arm extends (for example, in a punch), then how it retracts, such as in the final position for a block or in a preparatory position for a punch. Next, the major muscles and joints connecting the arm to the torso will be discussed.

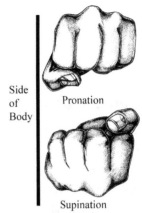

Side of Body

Pronation

Supination

Pronation vs. supination of the wrist.

Muscles and Joints Involved in Moving the Wrist

The wrist has two major positions (using the pivot joint of the radius and ulna), fully pronated and fully supinated. Pronation is when the wrist is fully rotated toward the body with the palm down and thumb rotated toward the body. This is the final wrist position in an extended straight punch (choku zuki). In order to fully pronate a wrist, the pronator teres muscle needs to be contracted while its antagonist, the supinator, needs to relax. Supination is when the wrist is fully rotated away from the body with the palm up and thumb away from the body. This is the final wrist position in soto ude uke. In order to fully supinate a wrist, the muscle that needs to be contracted is the supinator, while its antagonist, the pronator teres, needs to relax.

Generally, in karate the wrist is kept parallel to the forearm; however, in some techniques the wrist needs to be bent upward or downward. Several sets of muscles in the forearm help to articulate the hand by flexing downward (flexion) or extending upward (extension). The extensor carpi radialis and the brachioradialis let the wrist extend if in a supinated position with the hand open. If in a supinated position with the fist closed, the extensor digitorum and anconeus are employed. To flex the wrist back toward the body as in a palm heel strike (taisho uchi), the extensor digitorum, extensor digiti minimi, and the extensor carpi ulnaris are used.

Bending and Extending the Elbow

Extending the arm distally away from the body involves straightening the arm. This requires the hinge joint of the elbow to move through a flexion or straightening movement. In turn, this requires the triceps brachii, located on the underside of the humerus, to contract and the biceps brachii to relax. The opposite is true during extension: the biceps brachii, located on the upper side of the humerus, contracts and the triceps brachii relaxes.

How Is My Arm Connected to My Trunk?

In order to extend the arm in a shomen position, as in a straight punch, or choku zuki, the arm is extended distally at a right angle from the

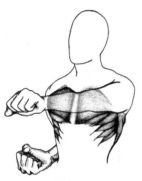

Major muscles used to connect the arm to the trunk.

torso. The major muscles that are involved, from arm to torso, are the anterior deltoids, pectoralis major, the latissimus dorsi, and the serratus anterior. At the same time, the muscles of the abdomen (rectus abdominis and external oblique) are also employed to allow the creation of intra-abdominal pressure (IAP; see chapter 14). To retract the elbow, as in the preparatory position for choku zuki and ushiro empi, the rear deltoid, trapezius, rhomboids, and latissimus dorsi are employed.

In short, the deltoids are used to pull and stabilize the shoulder joint, the pectoralis major pushes the shoulder girdle outward, and the latissimus dorsi and the serratus anterior contract the shoulder girdle downward, connecting the arm to the trunk. The trapezius and rhomboids pull the shoulder girdle backward toward the spine. As you are performing these techniques, it is important to be aware of the way these muscles articulate the skeleton. This means that in extending the arm distally from the body, one must only contract the muscles needed for extension. The muscles not involved in this motion need to be completely relaxed.

In the hanmi position, with elbow one fist from the hip (either straight or bent), as in soto ude uki or gedan barai, the major muscles employed are the middle deltoids, the pectoralis major, the latissimus dorsi, the serratus anterior, trapezius, and rhomboids. The number of muscles employed in this position makes it clear why this position is so stable and connected to the body. In a hanmi position, with a raised elbow, as in age uke or kizami zuki, the trapezius is also employed. But there is some loss of the contribution of the pectoralis major, which is why age uke is somewhat weak relative to a force from the left or right.

Muscles and Joints Involved in Moving the Lower Body

Following this general explanation of joints and muscles, we can now explain how these can relate to movements useful in karate, leg techniques in particular. First, we will see how the leg extends in a kick or the driving rear leg in zenkutsu dachi. Next we'll discuss the retraction or bending of the leg, as in the load position for a kick or the bent leg in a stance. We will then examine the major muscles and joints involved in how the leg then connects to the hip, which will in turn drive the body center forward and add power to the technique.

Flexion of the Ankle

In karate, the ankle joint can be either plantar flexed (flat relative to the shin) or dorsiflexed (pulled back toward the shin). In addition, the ankle can be supinated, as in the final position for yoko geri keage.

The major muscles involved in plantar flexion of the ankle are the gastrocnemius, soleus (calf), tibialis posterior, fibularis brevis and longus, flexor hallucis longus, flexor digitorum longus, and plantaris. When performing mae geri, the toes also need to be pulled back. This is achieved by relaxing the flexor hallucis longus and contracting the extensor halluces longus. The major muscles involved in dorsiflexion are the tibialis anterior, extensor digitorum longus, extensor hallucis longus, and peroneus tertius.

Extension and Flexion of the Knee

The primary muscles involved in the straightening of the knee joint are the quadriceps, including the vastus lateralis, rectus femoris, and the vastus medialis. The primary muscles involved in the flexion of the knee joint (bending the leg) are the hamstrings, semimembranosus, biceps femoris, and semitendinosus. As with the biceps-triceps antagonist relationship, the quadriceps-hamstrings are in the same relationship. Therefore, in order to extend the leg quickly, the quadriceps need to be shortened and the hamstrings must be completely relaxed.

Connection to the Hip

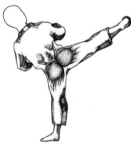

Major muscles used in yoko geri kekomi.

In karate we often mistakenly refer to the hip as a moving joint. The hip girdle does not move. Rather, it is the head of the femur in the ball-and-socket joint in the hip that completes the movement. It is the muscles that connect the legs to the hips that move the hip. This type of movement is akin to having two toothpicks one inch apart in the base of a potato and pushing and pulling on the toothpicks so that the potato rotates.

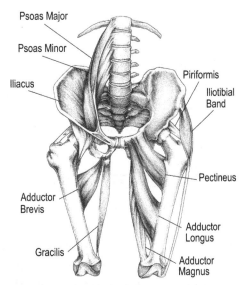

Major muscles used in the hip.

To move the leg directly behind the body (as in ushiro geri or the back leg of zenkutsu dachi), the gluteus maximus must be innervated and, to a lesser degree, the gluteus medius on the side. To lift the leg out to the side in a yoko geri kekomi position, the gluteus medius and to some extent the gluteus maximus are primarily used. As the leg moves to a yoko geri keage position, the gluteus medius and the tensor fascia latae come into play. The gluteus medius and the tensor fascia latae are often called the abductors. The leg is lifted into a mae geri position with the help of the iliopsoas, which is made up of the psoas major, the liacus, and the quadriceps. The rectus femoris and satoris can also be used to a lesser degree. Muscles that allow the leg to move inward are the adductor brevis, adductor longus, adductor magnus, and the gracilis, all collectively known as the adductors. The psoas major and iliacus muscle can also innervate an upward tilting of the hip.

The psoas major is an interesting muscle since it connects from the spine to the front of the hip. In mice, this muscle is composed of fast type II twitch fibers, a type of muscle that completes fast-twitch actions. However, in humans it contains both slow and fast-twitch fibers. This could be part of the reason why the hip motion in karate takes a long time to develop: the fast-twitch fibers in this deep hip muscle need to be developed over time.

One important consideration for any techniques involving the leg and hip muscles is that it is paramount to spend time stretching these muscles. For this reason, a deep understanding of the agonist-antagonist relationship is important.

Dynamic and Static Contraction

Finally, we should note the difference between dynamic and static muscles. As we have discussed previously and will discuss in depth in chapter 13, it is important to reconcile both acceleration and speed with mass, two seemingly opposing concepts, to create force or momentum. Therefore, it is also important to understand not only the agonist-antagonist relationship in terms of creating the movement of the limb toward the target, but also the stabilizing muscles during the impact phase of the technique. Of particular importance during the impact phase are the torso muscles involved in intra-abdominal pressure (IAP) and the associated core muscles used in the final stabilization at the finish of the technique, such as the latissimus dorsi in choku zuki.

It is crucial, then, to know what muscles are used in each technique (only use those muscles and relax all others) and the order in which they need to be fired. This can only be achieved through constant practice of karate.

References

Link, N., and L. Chou. *The Anatomy of the Martial Arts: An Illustrated Guide to the Muscles Used in Key Kicks, Strikes, and Throws.* Berkeley, CA: Ulysses Press, 2011.

Marieb, E. N., and K. Hoehn. *Human Anatomy and Physiology.* 9th ed. New York: Pearson, 2012.

CHAPTER 12

How the Body Works: Balance

Balance and the center of gravity are central to locomotion and therefore central to karate training. In some respects, walking could be defined as organized falling, where you unbalance forward and your feet catch up to prevent the fall. Therefore, understanding the center of gravity and being able to control one's body center provides a key to both efficient movement from one position to another and to unbalancing an opponent. This chapter will discuss the concepts of center of gravity and balance, along with their effects on equilibrium, stability, and mobility.

Center of Gravity

The center of gravity (CG) is defined as the balance point of the body. It is the single point where all forces on the body equal zero. This means that in all three axes (top to bottom, left to right, and front to back), the forces acting on the body are zero and all rotary

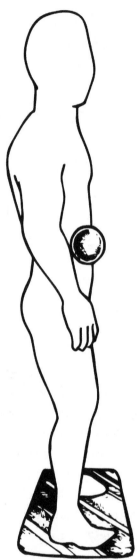

Illustrated as a ball, this diagram shows where the center of gravity is located.

forces (forces coming from the muscles) are balanced. One way to think about this is to imagine a ball placed at this point (center of the body). If you look through a camera toward the center of the person and move the camera in any direction while still looking toward the person's center, the ball will not shift position from your perspective.

The other important point about the CG is that if the body shifts in terms of shape or posture, the CG will also shift in location. For example, the CG of a person standing at attention in heisoku dachi is located a few inches below the belly button and a few inches inside the person. If they lift both arms upward so they are straight out in front, the CG will shift forward a few inches. Thus, the CG changes depending on what different parts of the body, called segments, are doing. In addition, depending on the shape of the body, the CG does not necessarily need to be inside the body (see the illustration in the next section).

With this in mind, the location of the CG will differ slightly depending on the shape, build, sex, and age of the individual. For example, a male and female's CG are approximately 57 percent and 55 percent of their standing heights, respectively.

Equilibrium, Stability, and Balance

Generally, when an object is at rest it is in equilibrium; this means that all forces acting on it are balanced. Therefore, the sum of all linear forces and all torques is equal to zero. However, not all objects at rest are equally stable. Someone standing on one foot in a balanced position will have less stability even though she is at equilibrium compared to when she is standing with both feet on the ground with the feet shoulder width apart.

An object has stable equilibrium when an effort to disturb it would require its CG to be raised. So if you have a brick lying on its side, you would have to lift the brick to disturb it. An unstable equilibrium involves the opposite: a slight disturbance will drop the object's CG to a lower point, normally from a smaller to a larger base of support. Imagine the same brick balanced on its edge. A slight disturbance would cause it to fall. In judo and karate, the concept of kuzushi, or unbalancing, means creating an unstable equilibrium. The idea is to push or pull an opponent to create an

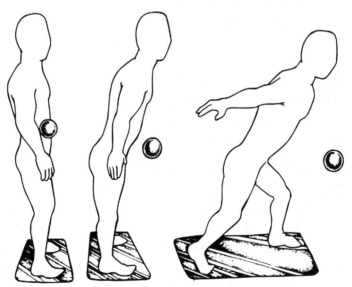

The center of gravity moves as the body changes position. In order to maintain balance, the center of gravity must remain within our base of support.

unstable equilibrium. Finally, a neutral equilibrium is when an object's CG is neither raised nor lowered when it is disturbed. This is part of the reason one moves in zenkutsu dachi without raising or lowering the hips. In this way, stability is not compromised.

We can achieve a more stable equilibrium by ensuring that our CG remains within our base of support. This is easier to do if we have a larger base of support. In practical terms, this means the farther apart our legs are, the more stable we will be. For example, we are much more stable in zenkutsu dachi compared to renoji dachi or heisoku dachi. One important consideration, since humans are bipedal, is that our base of support is normally a band between the feet. This explains the weak angles of different stances. Kiba dachi, for instance, is very stable in the side-to-side direction, but unstable front to back. This is because the base of support is longest from foot to foot, so it is easier to keep the CG within the base of support when resisting lateral forces.

Another way to increase stability is to make use of the vertical center of gravity. Simply put, it is easier to move the CG away from the base of support if there is a longer lever. If the CG is low to the ground, then it has to move along a much steeper angle to become unstable. However, if the CG is high up, then it is much easier. To take a simple example, think about cutting a lock. Bolt cutters with a longer handle are easier to maneuver because they have a longer lever, while short-handled bolt cutters are much harder to use because of the short lever.

Mass and friction can also jeopardize stability. Generally, it is harder to destabilize a larger mass than a smaller mass. Friction, or the force resisting movement due to contact with the ground (think slippery ice versus rough concrete), is important in that the amount for friction that is required to destabilize an object is directly related to the size of the base of support and the nature of the surface. For example, the greater the contact with the ground, the harder it is to destabilize the object.

Other Factors?

Humans, being bipedal, spend a lot of their time moving and adjusting their body parts to the type of equilibrium required by the task at hand. They do this by adjusting their center of gravity. This is natural and one of our basic motor skills. While all of the aforementioned factors play a role in balance, there are additional factors.

Physiologically, our eyes govern our perception of balance. If we are in a stable environment with unstable visuals (e.g., on a stable bridge but crossing a fast river), our sense of balance may be disturbed. In addition, when the semicircular canals in our ears are affected by colds and the like, our balance can also be affected.

Principles of Stability

According to Hamilton et al. (see under references), there are nine basic principles of stability:

1. The lower the CG, the greater the body's stability.

2. Greater stability is obtained if the base of support is widened in the direction that force is being applied.

3. For maximum stability, the line from your center of gravity to the floor should intersect the base of support at a point that will allow the greatest range of movement. Ideally, this will be in the direction of the forces causing motion.

4. The greater a body's mass, the greater will be its stability.

5. The most stable position of a person is one in which the backbone and CG lies in a vertical line centered over the base of support.

6. The greater the friction between the supporting surface and the parts of the body in contact with it, the more stable the body will be.

7. A person has better balance when moving under difficult circumstances when the vision is focused on stationary objects rather than on disturbing stimuli.

8. There is a positive relationship between one's physical and emotional states and the ability to maintain balance under difficult circumstances.

9. Regaining equilibrium is based on the same principles as maintaining it.

The Link between Stability and Mobility

Finally, there exists an inverse relation between stability and mobility. As noted above, walking can be thought of as controlled organized falling, where the CG is shifted forward beyond the base of support, creating instability. In order to compensate, the leg swings through to reestablish that base. The net result is forward movement.

Therefore, practitioners should develop the ability to control changes from stability to instability and back at will. In karate this is often referred to as controlling your center. In short, to increase speed at the start of a movement, the CG should be as close to the edge of a base of support as possible, while a quick stop requires a large base of support. This is exemplified by zenkutsu dachi, where the front ankle is tucked under the body, creating a large bend through the front knee. This has the effect of shifting the CG close to the edge of the base of support under the front leg.

Finally, it is important to stress the fundamental ability in karate to control one's center of gravity. The simplest way is to maintain a straight perpendicular posture relative to the floor. Small shifts in the torso, such as moving the torso away from an angle that is perpendicular to the floor, can result in marked shifts in the CG, making the body center and thus balance much harder to control. It is useful to imagine the body center and the CG as the same thing. Do everything possible to keep your posture straight and move your CG and body center together as one unit. This way you can rotate and move in a controlled fashion. For many, this is the single hardest thing to master.

References

Hamilton, N., W. Weimar, and K. Luttgens. *Kinesiology: Scientific Basis of Human Motion.* 12th ed. New York: McGraw-Hill, 2011.

Marieb, E. N., and K. Hoehn. *Human Anatomy and Physiology.* 9th ed. New York: Pearson, 2012.

Nakayama, M. *Dynamic Karate: Instruction by the Master.* Tokyo: Kodansha International, 1966.

Okazaki, T., and M. V. Stricevic. *The Textbook of Modern Karate.* New York: Kodansha International, 1984.

Otaki, T., and D. F. Draeger. *Judo: Formal Techniques.* Tokyo: Tuttle Publishing, 1983.

CHAPTER 13

Biomechanics: How Do I Hit Something Hard?

Kinesiology is the study of human movement; it includes physiology, mechanics, and psychology. It can be applied to biomechanics, strength and conditioning, sport psychology, rehabilitation, and sport science (*1*). Master Nakayama began reconciling traditional karate with modern kinesiology, which led to a more scientific approach to the performance and teaching of karate techniques (*2, 3*).

This chapter will provide a brief introduction to the application of kinesiological principles to karate. Body structure and articulation will be introduced first. The basic principles of biomechanics and how they can be applied to karate in the context of the question of "How can I hit something harder?" will also be discussed.

Body Structure According to Biomechanics

The human body consists largely of a central trunk or core and four limbs. In terrestrial bipedal animals, two of these limbs, the legs, are used for locomotion, while the other two, the arms, are used to articulate the environment or objects. Additionally, humans have an endoskeleton consisting of 206 bones that are articulated by a complex set of agonist-antagonistic muscle groups.

Each limb has the same three general structures. The structure closest to the trunk is a stylopod (humerus/femur), which connects the hip/shoulder girdle through the ball-and-socket joint of the shoulder to the hinge joint of the elbow. The zeugopid (radius, ulna/tibia, fibula) connects the hinge joint of the elbow to the wrist bones. Furthest from the body, the autopod (carpals/tarsals) makes up the hand and foot.

From a biomechanical standpoint, the body can be viewed as a flexible core cylinder with smaller articulated cylinders, one for each of the stylopod, zeugopid, and autopod, representing each limb.

Action of Muscles, Tendons, Ligaments, and Skeleton

The endoskeleton of the human body is articulated by a complex set of muscles that are connected to the bones by tendons. Ligaments hold the individual bones together.

As we discussed in the previous chapter, muscles are set up in groups so that they are in an agonist-antagonist relationship to each other. They are set up this way because muscles can only shorten; therefore, all articulation of the skeleton is through the shortening of the muscles or due to the effect of gravity (4).

This means that the body is constructed of a series of levers (1). A lever is defined as a rigid object used on an axis to multiply either the mechanical force (effort) or the resistance force (load) applied to it. The efficiency of a lever is called the mechanical advantage (*MA*). *MA* can be calculated by dividing the effort arm (*EA*) by the resistance arm (*RA*) (*MA = EA/RA*). Simply put, the greater the *MA* the less effort required. There are three components to a lever: the axis

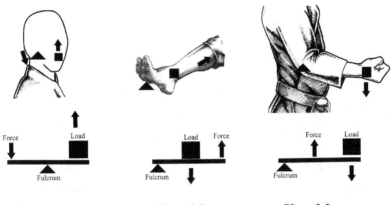

Class 1 Lever   Class 2 Lever   Class 3 Lever

Different levers of the human body.

(or fulcrum), the recessive load (or weight), and the force (effort). It is the location of these components that determines mechanical advantage. Location of the fulcrum makes levers either first, second, or third class. Therefore, levers can be first, second, or third class.

First-class levers are when the fulcrum is located between the force and load. In this case, there is no mechanical advantage. Second-class levers have the load between the fulcrum and the force. This means that the force lever arm is always greater than the load lever arm. These types of levers give a mechanical advantage. Third-class levers are when the force is applied between the fulcrum and the load. This means that the load lever arm is always greater than the force lever arm. These types of levers provide a mechanical advantage of less than one (this represents a seesaw with two people of equal weight on either end where the force in equals the force out). It is interesting to think that many of the levers in the human body are third-class levers that have a disadvantage when it comes to effort and load. In short, it is like having a seesaw where one person is much closer to the center fulcrum than the other. Simply put, the person who is closer will have more work to do in lifting the person who is farther away. However, this is only true when one considers the movement at the end of the lever. Simply put, using third-class levers allows a small arc of motion proximally at the muscle insertion point but creates larger, faster movement at the far end of the arm (i.e., the person at the long end of the seesaw will move much farther and faster than the person on the short end). This makes the use of class-three levers very efficient in terms of human motion and karate.

Motion Types

In basic biomechanics, two types of motion are prevalent. The first is linear motion. This is motion in a straight line, from one point to another. Linear motion uses linear Newtonian physics. A slight variation of linear motion is curvilinear motion, which is in a straight line but takes a curved path. The second type is angular motion. This is when all parts of the body move through the same angle, in the same direction and at the same time, but do not move through the same distance. This type of motion is governed by rotational physics.

Biomechanics and the Great Conundrum of Karate

Physics, especially Newtonian physics, explains a lot about how karate works. Variables such as speed, velocity, acceleration, force, and momentum (both linear and angular), and the relationship among them, can be directly applied to everyday training. In addition, gravity, center of gravity, base of support, and whether the motion is active (generated by muscle contraction) or passive (movement is caused by another factor, such as gravity) also play important roles and should be considered.

Speed and velocity are defined as distance divided by time. The difference between the two is that velocity has directionality (vector) associated with it. Both can be defined using the following formula: $s = d/t$ or $v = d/t$, where s = speed, v = velocity, d = distance, and t = time.

Acceleration is measured as the change in speed divided by change in time in a particular direction. This allows a measure of how much velocity is increasing over a given time. Generally, if acceleration is positive, then the object is speeding up; if acceleration is decreasing, the object is slowing down toward or away from an object.

Force is a measure of the influence on an object to undergo change. For example, to move an object, a force needs to be applied that is greater than the amount that can push back (due to friction, or mass). Force is equal to acceleration times mass and is represented by the formula $F = ma$, where F = force, m = mass, and a = acceleration.

Momentum is a measure of how much energy carried in a moving object can be transferred to the target. It is defined by $p = mv$, where p = momentum, m = mass, and v = velocity.

The final concept is that of kinetic energy, or Ek. Kinetic energy is the energy an object possesses due to its motion. It is defined by the formula $Ek = \frac{1}{2}mv^2$, where kinetic energy is equal to half the mass of the hitting object multiplied by the velocity of the hitting object squared.

In practical martial art terms, force and momentum are the "weight of the hit." For example, a statement like, "He hit like a train" would indicate a large amount of force and momentum being delivered to the target. Kinetic energy would be the penetrating energy that is absorbed by the object. The feeling of "Man, he hit me and I felt it explode out of my back" is an example of a hit with high kinetic energy.

The important points about these latter three formulas are the relationships between fast movement or acceleration and mass. Both of these elements need to be maximized to create the greatest possible momentum or force that can be applied to a target. This is one of the great conundrums of karate. A karateka needs to throw a fully relaxed technique (free from antagonistic muscle intervention), but then maximize the full body mass at the point of impact rather than just the mass of the attacking limb. As martial artists, we are taught to relax throughout the technique. This allows us to greatly speed up the technique. However, if we hit with a completely relaxed arm or foot, we will lose the crucial component of having the full body weight behind the technique. Conversely, if we "muscle" the technique (by using both the agonist and antagonist muscles together) we will greatly slow the technique, decreasing its impact. Either way, we want to find a way to maximize *both* speed and mass at the point of impact.

This then raises the question of which is more important to develop, mass or speed? By comparing the momentum and kinetic energy formulas, and testing them with some simple numbers, we can see an interesting trend (shown in the table below). If we have an object that weighs 10 kg (22 lb) and it is moving at a velocity of 10 meters per second (m/s), which is about 30 ft/s, we will have a momentum of 100 kg m/s and a kinetic energy of 500 Joules (J). (A Joule is just the standard unit of measurement for kinetic energy. It is equal to 1 kg m^2/s^{-2}, but you don't need to know that. What is important is to notice the relationship between mass, velocity, and kinetic energy, and that the bigger momentum and the bigger kinetic energy, the better.) If we then increase the mass by 50 percent to 15 kg and leave the velocity at 10 m/s, the momentum will increase by 50 percent to 150 kg m/s, and the kinetic energy will increase by 75 percent to 750 J. If we now reduce the mass back to 10 kg but increase the velocity by 50 percent to 15 m/s, we now get a momentum increase of 50 percent to 150 kg m/s, but our kinetic energy more than doubles to 1,125 J. This is illustrated in the table below. As it shows, by working on both mass and speed we can increase our momentum; however, to develop our penetrating power it is more useful to work on speed. Therefore, based on this relationship, it is obvious that as good martial artists we need to concentrate on developing both speed and mass. We will now spend some time discussing the development of each.

	Starting	Increase mass by 50%	Increase speed by 50%
Starting mass m (kg)	10 kg	15 kg	10 kg
Starting velocity v (m/s)	10 m/s	10 m/s	15 m/s
Momentum $p = mv$ (kg m/s)	100 kg m/s	150 kg m/s	150 kg m/s
Percentage increase in momentum compared to starting mass and speed		50%	50%
Kinetic energy	500 J	750 J	1,125 J
Percentage increase in kinetic energy compared to starting mass and speed		75%	112.5%

How Do I Become Faster?

To get faster, the practitioner works on several areas. In short, they are the relaxation of the antagonistic muscles, the building of fast-twitch muscle, flexibility, correct paths of motion, and the good use of hips or the body center.

Relaxation of Antagonistic Muscles

In order to make speedy movements, it is vital that only those muscles actually involved in the movement be innervated. As we stated earlier in this chapter, since muscles can only pull, all muscles are set up with an agonist and an antagonist, like a pair of counter springs. Therefore, any innervation of the antagonistic muscle will fight the movement of the agonist and thus slow down the movement. For example, if you are trying to straighten your arm, you need to completely relax your biceps while innervating your triceps. Any innervation of the biceps will result in a slowing of the movement. It can be seen in the graph

Relax all muscles but those that are important

Flexability
Static - lengthen + hold
Passive - Partner
Active - str, unassisted
Ballistic - Bouncing X
Dynamic - Controlled
PNF - stretch + contract

Efficienty of Neuromuscular Pathways

Do + ECONOMY of Motion
- Direct Pathway
- Repitition so muscles Know which order to fire

Translation
$P = MV + EK = \frac{1}{2} mv^2$
Step, shift, jump - Tobi
Oi   Yori (slide)
orayumi   Okuri (front)
ashi   Sugi (back)
- shift w/o moving feet

Key Shift
Bend in Knee!

Speed!
Use of Hips

Elevation
- drop 9.8 m/s/s
- Lift both Legs

Rotation

BIG PROBLEM
- if Max Velocity is achieved then mass = Ø!
∴ P = Ø + EK Ø!
How Couple??

Vibration
Intra Abdominal Pressure
"Connection"

Direct   Reverse
hip   arm   arm   hip
same   opposite

Concept of I (other side)
t = same
B moves faster!
- Foot feel to move hips.
- Axis Point

However, Body Center must move Forward!

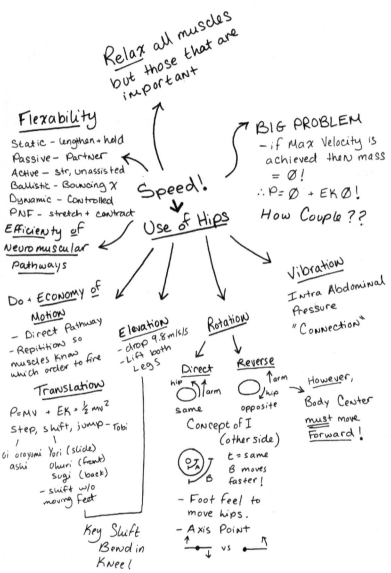

Different ways a karate practitioner can maximize speed.

showing speed vs. distance of a technique that as our limb moves over a certain distance to the striking surface, we will build speed; however, "muscling" the technique will cause us to fire the antagonist muscles, forcing the technique to slow down and

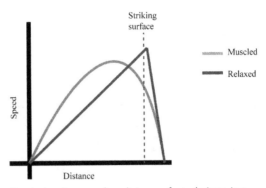

Graph showing speed vs. distance of a technique. In a relaxed technique (dark line), the speed increases until the target is hit. In a muscled technique (light line), the technique is slowing as the target is hit. (Adapted from Schmeisser, 1994.)

in fact be in a state of deceleration compared to when we hit the target versus a state of acceleration and therefore developing greater speed in our relaxed state.

When thinking of an isolated set of muscles, such as those involved in the biceps/triceps relationship, this process is fairly simple. But when thinking about a complex movement such as oi zuki that requires stepping the body forward into choku zuki and all of the subtle movements that result in hip vibration, the focus of relaxation is no longer simple. However, the fact is that even in this case, only muscles involved in forward motion need to be working. The simplest way to work on this is to break down each movement, study the muscles being used, and determine if that muscle needs to be flexing at that time in the movement. Then work on relaxing unneeded muscles, and step by step the movement will become more fluid and relaxed.

It is also important to point out that one needs to be relaxed at the beginning of any movement. From kamae, or ready position, every muscle should be relaxed, and there should only be enough tension in the body to hold the posture in place. Any excess tension will need to be relaxed before the body can go into motion, and this limits speed.

Building Fast-Twitch Muscle

In the body, there are several different types of muscle fibers: the type I, or slow oxidative (SO); the type IIA, or fast oxidative/glycolytic (FOG); and the type IIX, or fast glycolytic (FG). Of these, the SO muscle fibers have a slow twitch speed and a relatively small twitch force but are very hard to fatigue. On the other hand, the FG muscle fibers have a fast twitch speed and a large twitch force but fatigue easily. The FOG muscle fibers are intermediary to these two types and have a fast twitch speed, medium twitch force, and are fairly hard to fatigue (5).

Individual muscle fibers are set at birth and can vary by race. This means that an individual cannot build new muscle fibers but can develop and increase the thickness of them. Therefore, an individual is genetically restricted in terms of the ratios of these three muscle fiber types. An individual can, however, develop one muscle fiber type in a muscle individually. For example, if someone has 50 percent SO and 50 percent FG fibers, he or she can work, through training, to develop one muscle fiber type over another, thereby developing the ratio of SO to FG in the total mass from 50/50 to 72/25 (5).

In order to develop speed, the practitioner needs to develop FG fibers. In general, lifting either a heavy weight with slow acceleration or lifting a lighter weight with fast acceleration can achieve this. This can make use of classical heavy weight training, plyometrics, agility drills, sprints, and medicine ball training.

Development of Flexibility

Flexibility refers to the lengthening of the muscles. Simply put, the longer the muscle can stretch, within reason, the greater the range of movement. In addition, flexibility helps with the counter-spring architecture of the muscles in that the antagonist is free and long enough to move through its range. Flexibility also helps prevent muscle pulls and strains.

There are many different forms of stretching (6). Ballistic stretching uses body weight to bounce into the stretch. This kind of stretching, however, has been shown to actually tighten up the muscle and can thus cause injury, and therefore it should not be practiced. Dynamic stretching uses controlled movements to take you to the range of your stretch. With active stretching, you assume a position and hold it using the agonist muscle. Many of the movements in yoga are based on active stretching (7). Passive/static stretching has you assume a position and use alternative limbs, a partner, or some other apparatus to hold the stretch. This type of stretching is very good for cooling down. In isometric stretching, the antagonist muscle is used to help facilitate the stretch. An example of this type of stretching is proprioceptive neuromuscular facilitation (PNF). To do this type of stretching, one sets into a position, then pushes against the stretch. For example, if you are stretching your hamstrings, push your leg down into the floor tensing the quadriceps for ten seconds, then relax, and you will be able to move farther into your hamstring stretch. This type of stretch develops muscle in the antagonist while developing the proprioceptors (the structure in the muscle that signals that a muscle is being stretched) as well as lengthening the agonist. Children should not do PNF or isometric stretching, as their bones and tendons are still developing.

In general, karate training makes use of active stretching through the use of deep and strong karate stances. This is very similar to yoga movements (e.g., the active stretching in warrior I is like the stretch in zenkutsu dachi shomen, and the stretch in warrior II is similar to zenkutsu dachi hanmi). In addition, the movements in kicks and punches are good dynamic stretches. A skilled instructor will lead a warm-up and cool-down to include elements of active, dynamic, passive, and (depending on the class) occasionally isometric stretching.

The Development of the Correct Paths and Timing of Motion

In order to have good speed, the movement must be efficient. The adage "the shortest distance between two points is a straight line" is especially true here, since distance in the correct direction is a key component of speed. Simply put, changing direction during a movement reduces speed because of the change in the vector of movement. The difference can be thought of as a ten-pin blowing ball rolling directly down the lane versus bouncing off lane bumpers. If two balls are moving at the same speed, the zigzagging one will take much longer to reach the end because it is traveling a longer distance. This concept needs to be applied to every part of the body. The attacking weapon needs to move along its vector, whether arc or straight line, directly toward the target, while the body center also needs to travel directly toward the target. Every joint articulation needs to happen in the correct sequence and direct the technique toward the target.

Developing this type of neuromuscular control requires the practitioner to pay close attention to which muscles fire and in what order. This requires careful analysis of body mechanics and ensuring that every part of the technique is helping the weapon move directly toward the target with no excess movement. Bruce Lee is often quoted as saying, "The object of martial arts is to simplify." Nowhere is this adage truer than here.

Once the analysis is complete, the practitioner needs to drill and repeat the movement numerous times. It is only through continued focused practice of correct movement that the right neuromuscular pathways can be entrenched. The correct movement literally needs to be drilled into the subconscious. This can take a long time, but as long as practitioners are aware of what they are doing and working toward it, they can achieve this.

Correct Recruitment of the Hips and Body Center

The hips are the origin of power in karate. They coordinate and provide the link among timing, control of body center, and the articulation of the upper and lower body for all techniques and movements in karate. There are several ways a practitioner can move the hips, including translation, elevation, direct and reverse rotation, and vibration. These five concepts will be discussed at length over the next three chapters.

By virtue of their location, the hips house the body center, often called seika tanden in karate. This point is located approximately two inches below the navel and two inches inside the body and should be constantly in the practitioner's mind when training. When striking a target, the body center should be in motion directly toward that target and never moving in any other direction, otherwise speed will be lost. Quite often, speed in karate means the speed of the hips and not the speed of the limbs.

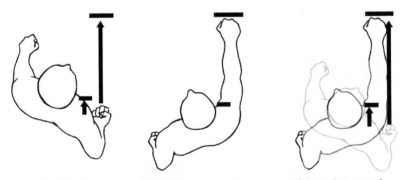

Hip and striking limb must move together through the duration of the technique. Left: preparatory position, showing the final positions of both the hip and fist (horizontal bars). Middle: hip and arm in the final positions at the conclusion of the technique. Right: both the hip and arm must move together throughout the entire technique. Because the hip moves a short distance, the arm must move very quickly.

The hips develop speed of technique since they function as a small lever. Simply put, they move a very short distance, while the limbs need to move a longer distance. Therefore, in order to hit a target while the body center and hips are in motion, the practitioner needs to work on timing of techniques in such a way that the striking weapon moves through its complete range of motion before the hips finish moving. This means that in a typical reverse punch, or gyaku zuki, the hips may move a total distance of one foot while the arm moves a total distance three times that. The arm, then, has to move three times as fast to have correct timing.

Practitioners often misinterpret speed as their hand or foot speed, but in actuality it is the speed of the hips that is important. In short, provided a practitioner has good timing between the hands or feet and hip, as described above, it can be argued that speed in karate should be defined by the speed of the hip. This just makes sense because the hip and body center are the fulcrum of all movement in karate; the faster the hip moves, the faster the limbs have to move to keep up. This can be difficult to develop and will take some time. The reason is that the muscles that work the hips are primarily slow oxidative muscles and are not often suited to fast-twitch movement.

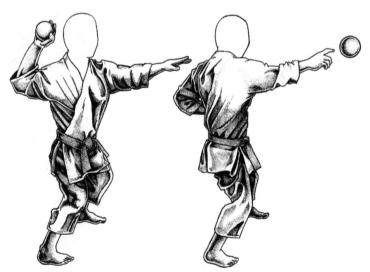

An example of the hip and arm working together, in this case throwing a ball.

How Do I Develop Mass?

While we have spent a great deal of time discussing speed and its importance, it is also vital to discuss mass as well. All of the formulas we have discussed above concerning speed (or acceleration) are multiplied, not added together to produce the resulting metric. This means that even if we generate as much speed as possible, if we do not couple it to our mass, then our resulting impact, whether measured in kinetic energy or momentum, will be reduced. After all, a million m/s multiplied by zero kilograms is still zero.

One of the central concepts of karate is the correct application of power, and this leads to one of the greatest conundrums in the martial arts. When and where to apply mass is key to correctly coupling mass and speed. Many beginners muscle their way through a technique; that is, they try throw as much muscle mass toward the target as possible. Unfortunately, this has the effect of simply innervating the antagonistic muscle group and slowing the technique down.

Here we will introduce methods to correctly apply mass to our techniques. The actual coupling will be introduced briefly here but will be discussed in depth in chapter 17. In short, there are several ways to increase mass: being bigger, moving the body center toward the target, proper final alignment of technique, correct connection of the upper and lower body, and correct coordination and timing of the technique.

Being Bigger

One of the easiest ways to increase mass is to simply be bigger. However, running out and eating a lot of fast food is not recommended. While you will acquire more mass, it will be in the form of fat and not muscle. Muscle is preferable to fat for two major reasons: first, muscle is much more dense compared to fat, and

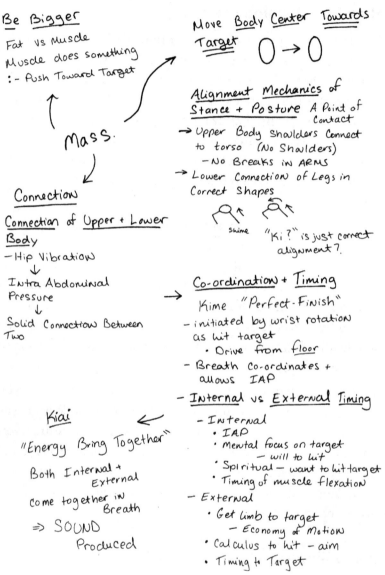

Be Bigger

Fat vs Muscle

Muscle does something

:- Push Toward Target

Mass.

Connection

Connection of Upper + Lower Body

- Hip Vibration
  ↓
Intra Abdominal Pressure
  ↓
Solid Connection Between Two

Kiai

"Energy Bring Together"

Both Internal + External

Come together in Breath

⇒ SOUND Produced

Move Body Center Towards Target O → O

Alignment Mechanics of Stance + Posture A Point of Contact

→ Upper Body shoulders connect to torso (No Shoulders)
  — No Breaks in ARMS
→ Lower Connection of Legs in Correct Shapes

shime   "Ki?" is just correct alignment?

Co-ordination + Timing

Kime "Perfect-Finish"

- initiated by wrist rotation as hit target
  • Drive from floor
- Breath Co-ordinates + allows IAP

- **Internal** vs **External** Timing

  - Internal
    • IAP
    • Mental focus on target
      — will to hit
    • Spiritual — want to hit target
    • Timing of muscle flexation

  - External
    • Get limb to target
      — Economy of Motion
    • Calculus to hit — aim
    • Timing to Target

Different ways a karate practitioner can maximize mass.

therefore the practitioner will gain more mass by acquiring more muscle. Second, fat does not contract; it is sessile, while muscle contracts, thus creating movement.

While gaining mass is a good thing, there is a trade-off in that the more mass one has, the harder it is to move the body quickly in a particular direction. This could be thought of as the time it takes a motorcycle to get up to speed compared to a train. The more massive train requires a large engine and a relatively long time to get its mass moving. This concept is called inertia. Thus, it is important for practitioners to make sure the amount of mass they build is proportional to their body frame. Moreover, regular explosive training, as well as regular stretching, as discussed above, is important. Therefore, simply building more mass is good but limited. It is better to concentrate on how to use the mass that one has more efficiently.

Move the Body Center toward the Target

As we discussed above, the body center is vital to all karate movement. In particular, the movement of the body center is critical to the development of our mass component. The body center, as a general rule, should always be in motion, and preferably accelerating, directly toward the target as the striking limb comes into contact with the target. This allows one's total body weight to be delivered to the target.

Students are often told that the hand and foot must move at the same time. People misinterpret this to mean that when stepping, the front foot needs to place as the hand finishes its rotation. I disagree with this interpretation because when the front foot places, the hips stop moving toward the target. This then removes the body weight and only allows the weight of the arm to be delivered to the target. An analogy could be driving a train, then stopping the train and throwing a stone that hits the target. Effectively, all of the momentum created by moving the body center toward the target is lost. My personal feeling is that the concept of hand and foot timing, especially when driving forward in oi zuki, refers not to the front leg, but rather to the straightening of the rear leg, which is in turn timed with the connection of the body (see below) and the limb hitting the target. Therefore, timing is critical.

One other important point is that the body center should never move away from the target, unless absorbing a technique when blocking. When throwing a jab, or kizami zuki, for example, practitioners often lean forward with their shoulders. This has the effect of moving the body center backward and in the direction opposite that of the punch. This causes a dramatic decrease in the potential mass that can be delivered to the target. Moreover, when techniques are delivered from a static position such as kiba dachi, it is important that the body center move toward the target within the limits of the construction of the stance. A perfect example is in the opening sequence of the kata Tekki shodan in Shotokan. The hips are turned as far as possible to the right following an elbow strike. The next sequence of movements—the preparatory position for the gedan barai (lower block) and the kagi zuki (hook punch)— need to have hip rotation toward the target in a piecemeal fashion as far as the constraints of the stance allows, not letting the knees buckle and thus losing the integrity of the stance. The hips often incorrectly move counter to the hook punch. The target is to the left, say, but the hips are moving in the opposite direction. One final example is the dynamic movement of any of the blocks that cross the body and involve a reverse hip rotation motion, such as gedan barai (lower block). If this technique is used to stop an opponent rather than deflect, then the hips need to be driven forward into the technique. This is discussed in more depth in chapter 16.

Alignment (Mechanics of Stance and Posture)

The next key element of mass is to create the most stable structure possible at the moment of impact. Many of the stances and postures developed in karate are designed to do just that. They provide a stable connection to the floor, good posture, and intra-abdominal pressure. The arms are well seated in the shoulder joint, and the technique is able to provide correct bracing for the impact the technique delivers.

In order to have good alignment, it is important to understand several things about the body. The first is that straight lines are good. Straight arms and legs form a straight line from the radius and ulna in the forearm to the humerus in the upper arm as well as the tibia and fibula in the shin to the femur in the upper leg. This means that no energy will dissipate through the elbow or knee. Straight also means not locked. If the limb is locked, then it will actually bend slightly backward at the elbow or knee, and again energy will get dissipated at the joint. In some ways this can be thought of as a stick holding up a leaning brick wall. If the stick is bent or bowed, it has a high probability of breaking, while a straight stick will be able to brace the wall much better. The second thing to understand is that right angles can be good. The right angle presents the strongest position for the biceps to keep the arm bent due to utilizing the maximum number of filaments interacting in the muscle. Therefore, if the technique requires a bend in the elbow, then a ninety-degree angle is best. The third point is to seat the ball joint of the femur or humerus into the hip or shoulder, respectively. This allows a solid connection to the trunk via the gluteus maximus and latissimus dorsi. By this setting of the hip and shoulder, the trunk can be connected using intra-abdominal pressure. This connection will be discussed in the next section.

Another important point about alignment is to make sure that the stance is braced correctly against the direction of force. While the body center moves toward the target, it is important to be able to brace against the target on impact. Newtonian physics says that when force is applied against a stationary object, the

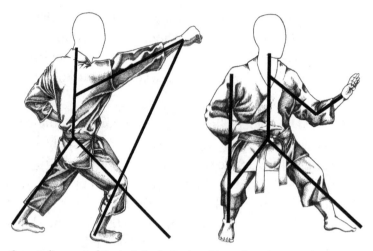

Correct alignment of the body in the final positions of two karate techniques. Left: zenkutsu dachi, oi zuki (lunge punch in front stance); right: kokutsu dachi, shuto uke (knife-hand block in back stance).

stationary object will push back with a force exactly equal to the force applied to it. The stances are structured in such a way as to provide the strongest bracing possible. Therefore, the stance must provide the correct posture and alignment. In addition, it is important that the karateka understand where the stance provides bracing. For example, zenkutsu dachi, or forward stance, provides bracing front to back and partial bracing side to side but is weak on a thirty-degree angle. Likewise, kiba dachi, or horse-riding stance, is strong side to side but weak front to back.

Connection of Upper and Lower Body

One of the key components of generating mass is to connect the striking limb to the driving leg. This is done through connecting the upper and lower body. In short, the connection is achieved through the correct application of intra-abdominal pressure (IAP), which allows the abdominal cavity to create a solid mass, a bridge between the upper and lower body. Provided the femur and humerus are seated correctly into the hip and shoulder as described above, there will be correct transmission of force from the floor to the striking limb. This concept is discussed in much more detail in chapter 14.

Coordination and Timing (Internal vs. External Timing/Breath)

One of the most important aspects of linking mass and speed is correct timing. This is achieved primarily through breath and effectively radiates from the center of the body. It is important to make initial contact with the target when the limb and body center are at maximum velocity and then lock the limbs down to create mass (see next section). Therefore, to hit something effectively, at the point of contact when the limb is at maximum velocity, the foot and driving leg must straighten and connect to the hip. The attacking limb must lock and seat into the shoulder. For example, if it is a punching arm, the wrist must rotate and the arm must connect into the shoulder joint. If it is a block, the elbow must connect to the hip. The coordination of the rotation of the wrist, the drive of the legs, and the correct application of IAP (see above and chapter 14) can be controlled from the center through breath. This coordination concept is discussed in more detail in chapters 17 and 18.

Other Elements

The way one impacts a target is also important in terms of the biomechanics of the impact time and the way the attack hits the target. Impacting a target is dealt with in chapter 18; however, there are two related concepts we need to examine here. The first is how long the fist is in contact with the target, and the second is the angle that can be used to maximize impact (8).

Impact Time

The amount of time that the striking limb remains in contact with the target depends on two major things. The first is the hardness of the weapon. The other is the hardness or softness of the target.

In most cases, the striking weapon should be made as hard or as heavy as possible when it strikes the target. This can be generally achieved by tightening the weapon at the point of impact. The classic example is tightening the fist as it comes into contact with the target. For most other weapons, we discussed how to tighten them for the point of impact in chapter 3. It is important, however, not to tighten the weapon too soon, as this will cause unnecessary innervation of the antagonistic muscles and will decelerate the limb. The weapon should be held in the correct shape throughout the path of movement, taking care not to loosen the hand so much that the fingers come completely loose. The weapon should tighten as it makes contact with the target an instant before the wrist rotates.

The target also plays an important role, especially in terms of how the karateka hits the target. In general, we are often advised to use a hard weapon to strike a soft target, and vice versa. This is popularized in many self-defense classes to prevent damage to the weapon. However, with correct conditioning, any weapon can be used to hit any target; the key is how long the weapon remains in contact with the striking surface. In karate there are three major ways to hit a surface: keage (snap), kekomi (thrust), and ate (smash). The dynamics of these are covered in depth in chapter 18. However, how they hit depends partly on how long the striking object remains in contact with the target. In general, impact force can be maximized on a hard surface, such as the face, compared to a soft target, such as the stomach. The blow tends to be more devastating to the target the shorter time it is in contact with the target. This concept is called impulse. Therefore, when a punch is delivered to a hard surface like the face, the attacking limb does not need to penetrate far into the target to deliver force. This, in turn, decreases the amount of time the attacking limb is in contact with the target. The opposite is true for a soft target like the stomach. The limb will hit and have to penetrate farther into the target, decelerating as it penetrates and increasing the time it is in contact with the target. This lessens the amount of impact force delivered to the target.

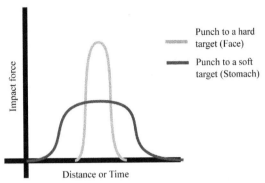

Graph showing the effect of impact force and distance or time when hitting a soft surface (dark line) vs. a hard surface (light line). Notice that the impact force is maximized when hitting a hard surface such as the face. The impact is less, but more sustained with the punch to a soft surface. This is the direct result of a phenomenon called impulse. (Adapted from Harrop, 2011.)

What Angle Do I Use?

Another important consideration is the angle at which two objects collide and how it pertains to the maximum amount of force that can be applied to an object. Generally, to hit a target with the maximum amount of force, the two surfaces need to collide at a ninety-degree angle to one another. Any angle that deviates from ninety degrees will result in less force being applied to the target. This concept is seen consistently in karate, where we have techniques designed to hit targets perpendicularly to their impact surface. For example, choku zuki, or straight punch, is designed to hit a surface parallel to the front of the body, while mawashi zuki, or roundhouse punch, is designed to hit a target at an angle, such as either side of the chin. The hook punch, kagi zuki, is designed to hit a surface at a right angle to the front of the body such as the side of head.

This same concept can be used for blocks where the practitioner will want to impact the target at an angle so that the impact is lessened on the forearm. The forearm is relatively small compared to the leg. Therefore, it is in the interest of the defender to ensure that a block happens at an angle other than ninety degrees to minimize the force transferred to the blocking limb.

Notes

1. N. Hamilton, W. Weimar, and K. Luttgens, *Kinesiology: Scientific Basis of Human Motion*, 12th ed. (New York: McGraw-Hill, 2011).
2. H. Cook, *Shotokan Karate: A Precise History* (England, 2001).
3. M. Nakayama, *Dynamic Karate: Instruction by the Master* (Tokyo: Kodansha International, 1966), 308.
4. D. L. Bartelink, "The Role of Abdominal Pressure in Relieving the Pressure on the Lumbar Intervertebral Discs," *J Bone Joint Surg* 39-B (1957): 718–725.
5. E. N. Marieb and K. Hoehn, *Human Anatomy and Physiology*, 9th ed. (New York: Pearson, 2012).
6. S. H. Kim, *Ultimate Flexibility: A Complete Guide to Stretching for Martial Arts* (Wethersfield, CT: Tuttle Press, 2004).
7. L. Chou and N. Link, *The Martial Artist's Book of Yoga: Improve Flexibility, Balance and Strength for Higher Kicks, Faster Strikes, Smoother Throws, Safer Falls, and Stronger Stances* (Berkeley, CA: Ulysses Press, 2005).
8. E. Schmeisser, *Advanced Karate-Do* (St. Louis: Focus Publications, 1994).

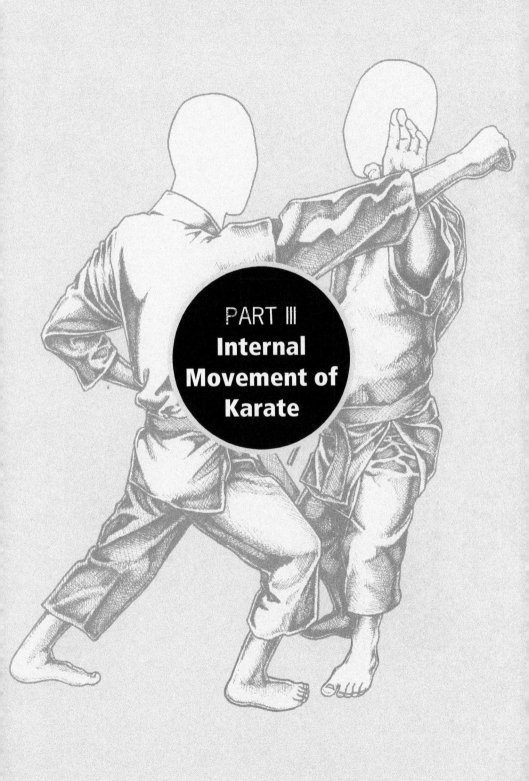

PART III
Internal Movement of Karate

CHAPTER 14

If I Jiggle My Hips, Do I Hit Someone Harder? Hip Vibration

Body vibration seems to be one of the most misunderstood concepts in karate-do. To some, it is a mystical way of generating energy from literally wiggling the hips; however, when rightly understood, it can become an important way to generate power. In my mind, hip vibration can be used for two purposes: First, it can connect the arms to the legs using a biological phenomenon called intra-abdominal pressure that will provide the mass component to any karate movement. This concept is often referred to in karate as kime. Second, used by itself, hip vibration allows the karateka to generate power without a lot of external movement.

An understanding of hip vibration can be gained through the study of the kata Tekki shodan in Shotokan or Po Eun in taekwondo. Though the kata has very little translational or rotational movement, the practitioner must generate power while keeping the integrity of the stance kiba dachi. Once the concept is understood, it can be applied to virtually every technique in karate.

So What Is Hip Vibration in Terms of Body Connection?

As we have already discussed, in order to hit something hard, the karateka needs to reckon with the seemingly paradoxical $F = ma$ formula. This formula states that the force that can be generated is a product of mass multiplied by acceleration. A similar paradox is involved in generating momentum as well ($p = mv$), where momentum is a product of mass multiplied by velocity. This paradox arises because in order to generate momentum or force, the practitioner needs to generate the maximum possible velocity or acceleration. This can only be done by relaxing the muscles and throwing the technique as fast as possible. The trade-off with this is that if the technique hits while all muscles are relaxed, they forgo the mass part of the equation, meaning that the impact will be weak since there will be no body weight behind the technique, just the weight of the attacking limb. Therefore, there needs to be a way to couple both speed and full body mass at one instant.

With this concept in mind, it is also important to develop a connection between the legs—connected, of course, to the floor—and the upper body. Again, if there is no connection between the two extremities, the practitioner will forgo the mass part of the aforementioned equations, and the potential momentum or force generated will diminish as a result.

Hip vibration is linked to both of these problems in a major way. Hip vibration comes about through a phenomenon called intra-abdominal pressure (IAP) (*1–3*).[6] Simply put, IAP is the flexion of the abdominal wall and the rectal muscles (in, not out), at the same time contracting the diaphragm downward to push the organs in the abdomen into the muscle walls to create a solid block.

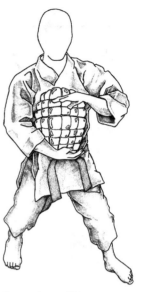

A useful analogy is a water balloon in a wire mesh bag. The bag is flexible and can bend and twist. However, if you apply pressure to the ends of the balloon (pushing the ends toward the center), the balloon will squeeze against the sides of the mesh bag and create a solid mass. In the body, a similar action connects the arms and legs.

The analogy of intra-abdominal pressure using a water balloon in a wire mesh bag as the viscera in the abdominal cavity.

Having the ability to form a solid mass between the legs and arms allows a direct coupling of upper and lower components of the body for an instant, creating the mass component of our force and momentum equations. Therefore, this concept should be tied to all karate translational and rotational hip movements. We will not be dealing with the coordination of these movements here, as they are the subject of chapter 17.

---

6. IAP is described by Norris (1993) as "contraction of the transversus abdominis, and to a lesser degree the internal and external obliques, will cause an increase in intra-abdominal pressure (IAP), when the glottis is closed. The muscles will pull on the rectus sheath and so compress the viscera. Compression of the abdominal contents forces them upward on to the diaphragm and separates the pelvis from the thoracic cage. The IAP will be greater if the breath is held after a deep inspiration, as the diaphragm is lower, and the comparative size of the abdominal cavity is reduced. By making the trunk into a more solid cylinder, axial compression and shear loads are reduced and transmitted over a wider area through the IAP mechanism."

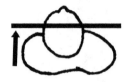

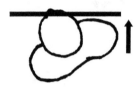

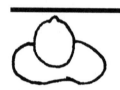

A top-down view of hip vibration. Bottom: the individual is standing square. Middle: the practitioner executes a punch with his right hand; the right hip drives forward accordingly, approximately one to two inches (to the black horizontal line). Top: upon the punch contacting the target, the wrist rotates. At the same time, the left leg drives off the floor and the torso compresses using IAP. This has the effect of instantaneously rotating the left hip so it is in line with the right (similar to slamming a door), and connecting the punch to the floor through the now-solid torso. Immediately, this position is relaxed and the body moves naturally back to the original position.

Can Hip Vibration by Itself Generate Power?

The short answer to this question is, sort of. It is fair to say that every karateka has gone through trainings where everybody stands in natural stance, or heiko dachi, and straight punches (choku zuki) to the count of the instructor. This drill is to develop understanding of hip vibration from a prone foot position. If you watch a class do this, you will see many variations of hip vibration, from no hip movement at all to wobbling from side to side.

Remember that in order to hit with power there needs to be some movement of the body center toward the target, even when the feet are prone. This principle must be observed, although, unfortunately, it is often not taught. Vibration, when it is isolated, is often taught as a short hip movement from side to side, rotating around a central axis. However, I disagree with this way of teaching the movement since students often fail to understand when it is explained this way and end up wobbling their hips because they do not understand the concept of intra-abdominal pressure and the connection it brings.

In my view, vibration is a product of the initiation of the movement through a drive from the attacking limb side, slightly causing the hip to rotate forward (middle figure). The abdomen compresses through IAP, while simultaneously the opposite driving leg pushes the opposite hip to be in line with the attacking limb hip (top figure). This couples a small one- to two-inch forward movement of the body center to IAP. Therefore, it is the quick application of relaxed hip movement, translating the body center slightly forward and coupled with IAP, that generates the vibrational movement of the hip, and not a conscious flopping movement of the hip.

As an example, if a practitioner is working on straight punch (choku zuki) from natural stance (heiko dachi), the vibrational movement is generated as follows: The practitioner initiates the movement with all muscles in the abdomen, shoulders, and arms relaxed. The hip on the same side as the punching hand is driven forward as far as the practitioner's hip flexibility allows while

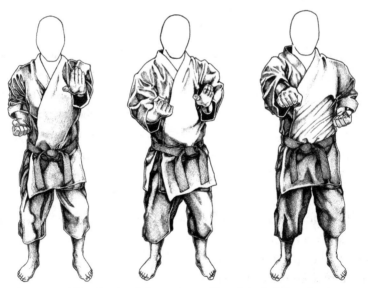

A front view of hip vibration. Left: starting position of the technique (analogous to the bottom figure in the previous illustration). Middle: initiation of a right choku zuki. Note that the right hip also drives forward with the punch (analogous to the middle figure in the previous illustration). Right: finish of the technique, where the left hip has driven forward as the body connects using IAP (analogous to the top figure in the previous illustration).

maintaining heiko dachi (normally just one to two inches). As the punch extends, the retracting hand comes back and the body is maintained in a relaxed state. At the point of contact, two things happen simultaneously: (1) The buttock on the same side as the retracting hand flexes, creating drive from the floor (shime) and driving the opposite hip forward slightly toward the target; and (2) the practitioner contracts his or her abdominals, squeezes the butt (from 1), and contracts the abdomen to create IAP, connecting the arms to the base. This has the effect of squaring the body to the front, except that the body center has translated a few inches forward from the original position and connects the feet to the punching hand, so that there is correct body alignment for the technique. Taking the example of our water-filled balloon in a mesh bag, if you twist it and then compress it quickly, it will untwist rapidly into its original orientation. Once the punch is completed, the abdomen relaxes and the body center resets to its initial position a few inches back.

In the first few movements of Tekki shodan, this concept is especially important. At no time should the body center be moving away from the target you are striking. Especially with respect to the hook punch, or kagi zuki, it is not uncommon to see the hips moving in the opposite direction, and thus the body center away from the target. As you move from the preparatory (cup-and-saucer)[7] position to the gedan barai to the kagi zuki, the hips should continue to rotate toward the target, and thus the body center moves in kind.

This concept can therefore be extrapolated and coupled into virtually every karate technique and every form of power generation, including translation, elevation, and both direct and reverse rotation (see next chapters). In addition, IAP plays a central part in kime, and also in the coordination of body movement.

---

7. Cup and saucer has one hand in the load position at the hip, while the other arm comes across the body with the hand sitting so that the bottom fist (tetsui) rests on top of the hand upturned hand on the hip.

Traditionally, there have been three major terms used to identify the means by which the body is able to generate power in karate. They are: body shifting, body rotation, and body vibration. The question may then be asked whether body vibration is the best term to describe the third means. Body vibration, as we have defined it here, is actually a combination of power generation though intra-abdominal pressure (IAP) and a small hip rotation, the major factor being the IAP.

Accordingly, one must question whether body vibration, as a term denoting a method of creating power, is useful. Based on our explanation above, the answer is simply no. Since what we term body vibration is nothing more than an extension of IAP (a tensing of the core muscles), I would prefer to use the term core compression, which indicates the role of IAP in the generation of power in karate movement.

Notes

1. P. R. Davis and J. D. G. Troup, "Pressures in the Trunk Cavities when Pulling, Pushing, and Lifting," *Ergonomics* **7** (1964): 465–474.
2. D. L. Bartelink, "The Role of Abdominal Pressure in Relieving the Pressure on the Lumbar Intervertebral Discs," *J Bone Joint Surg* **39-B** (1957): 718–725.
3. C. M. Norris, "Abdominal Muscle Training in Sport," *Br J Sp Med* **27** (1993): 19–27.

CHAPTER 15

Hit Them Like a Steam Train: Using Body Shifting to Generate Translational Power

Body shifting is a way to generate power from the body center by shifting the hips in a linear way. This can be in a vector either parallel to the floor, which is called translation, or perpendicular to the floor, which is known as elevation. In physics, body shifting can be described by the formula for momentum: $p = mv$, where p = momentum (measured in kg m/s), m = mass, and v = velocity. This says essentially that the faster you move a big object along a vector, the more momentum you will create. In particular, this type of movement can take the form of oi ashi (stepping) or yori ashi (shifting). In order to achieve any form of translational movement, you need to purposely unbalance yourself in the direction you want to travel. If you are in a perfectly balanced position, you are not moving. Therefore, by "organized falling," you can move forward.

Generally, for translation, the muscle propelling the limbs along that linear vector produces speed. In elevation, by contrast, especially when dropping the body center from a higher to a lower position, speed can also be produced by gravity. In addition, sometimes the practitioner can generate power by using elevation and translation simultaneously. Examples are fairly numerous in the kata, but the first movement in Bassai Dai (moving from attention, or heisoku dachi, to crossing stance, or kosa dachi), which requires both a step and a drop, is especially typical. Therefore, as with all hip power generation, more than one type is often applied simultaneously.

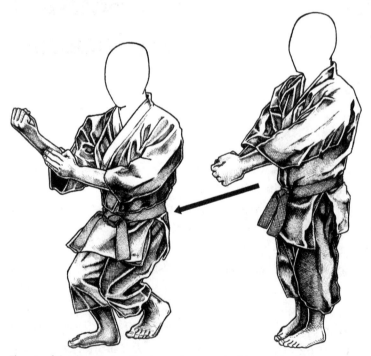

The use of the drop in elevation to create power. In this case, the first movement of the kata Bassai Dai.

Types of Translation and Elevation

There are several major types of translational and elevational movement. Especially prevalent movements are stepping, shifting, and jumping. Note that all of these, while having clear translational movement, can also incorporate elevational movement in both the upward and downward directions as well.

Stepping

Oi ashi, or stepping, refers to moving one foot to another position to move the body center in a particular direction. It can be in any direction as long as the front foot and rear foot are switched with each iteration. Examples of this include oi zuki, or stepping punch, where the practitioner drives off the front leg to push the rear leg through to the front, thus driving the hips forward. In the illustration below, the practitioner is stepping forward from left zenkutsu dachi to right zenkutsu dachi while punching with the right hand. It is important to note that, as with all translational motion elements of rotation, elevation and vibration may be incorporated.

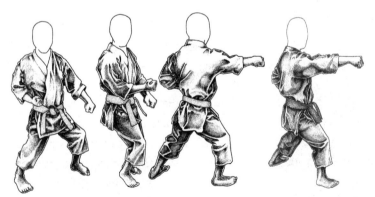

A sequence showing the progression of motion through oi zuki, or lunge punch, as it primarily uses body shifting to generate power. Note the elements of core compression (hip vibration) throughout the motion of this technique (analogous to what is described in chapter 14).

Dynamics of Oi Ashi

Stepping can vary dynamically depending on the tension of the initial stance (see chapter 5 for an explanation of stance tension). If the practitioner is moving from one outside-tension stance to another outside-tension stance (e.g., zenkutsu/kiba/kokutsu dachi to zenkutsu/kiba/kokutsu dachi), the overall feeling is to switch the tension from an outside-push feeling to a compression or squeeze from the adductors to compress the legs together using the hips as a fulcrum. This flows naturally to an expansion out to the final position where the feet grab the floor due to the outside tension. If the practitioner is stepping forward from one inside-tension stance to another inside-tension stance (e.g., Sanchin/Hangetsu dachi to Sanchin/Hangetsu dachi), the tension to create the initial compression is already there, so the relevant leg is simply released. The stance compresses and the legs come together using the hips as a fulcrum. Once the legs flow past each other, the stance starts to expand, and this time when the traveling foot makes contact with the floor, the feet grab the floor by applying outside tension as they move into the final position of the stance.

This feeling of contraction and expansion is important for the overall dynamic feeling of the movement, but the driving leg determines the directionality. Using a simple case of zenkutsu dachi to zenkutsu dachi, the step forward is initiated by the "hips" rotating slightly so that the rear-leg hip moves forward. Note that actually the legs and feet initiate all external movement by pushing off the ground. But it is easier to coordinate if the movement is thought of only in terms of the hip. This movement of the hip causes three things to happen simultaneously: (1) the feeling of outward tension is switched to inward tension in both feet; (2) the rear leg's heel lifts off the floor, initiating a push in the rear calf muscle; and (3) the front anchoring leg starts to pull the individual forward. This then initiates the adductors to squeeze the legs together, while the front leg pulls the body on top of it and the rear leg squeezes to the center as fast as possible. Next, as the legs pass each other and the front leg (now rear) starts to straighten and drive the body center forward more quickly, the rear leg (now front) simply swings forward to add momentum to the movement. Once at the right distance to hit the target, the new rear leg straightens, and simultaneously the abdominal region contacts through intra-abdominal pressure (see chapter 14). This snaps the hips to the correct half-face (hanmi) or full-face (shomen) position, connecting the hand technique to the driving leg and the floor. As long as this connection is achieved, it is relatively unimportant when the new front leg connects to the floor. Ideally, this should be at either the same time or a split second after the rear leg and abdominal region connect. This feeling of outward expansion is continued through the feet as they grab the floor. It is important to note here that while there is an outside tension in the feet with respect to the floor, the hips should remain supple and flexible after the initial connection.

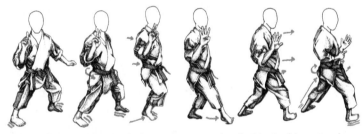

A sequence showing individual movement associated with oi ashi, or stepping techniques.

This same feeling arises when stepping backward. This time the movement is initiated by contracting the hip in the same way as above, with the rear-leg hip pushed slightly forward. The rear leg is anchored and pulls through the heel of the rear foot, squeezing the legs together. Squeezing through the adductors drags up the front leg. Note that the quadriceps is not the focus of movement here, as it will tend to lift the hip upward as the movement takes place. As the front leg swings backward and passes the opposite leg, the buttocks must contract quickly to swing the leg to increase momentum. Meanwhile, the opposite leg becomes the driving leg, pushing the body center backward. Connection of the abdominals is based on when the rear leg connects to the floor.

No matter the stances or the direction of the step, it is important that the driving leg have the feeling of being well connected to the floor and driving upward. This means that the practitioner must have the feeling of keeping the heel of the driving leg attached to the floor. This can be difficult depending on ankle flexibility. The feeling of an upward connection from the floor to the hip is called "shime" and is characterized by the sense that the femur is driving upward and into the buttocks.

Shifting either the front leg or the rear leg toward the center of the body on the initiation of a step in zenkutsu dachi (double stepping) can be a problem, as it is both inefficient in generating power and alerts the opponent to the attack due the double movement of the leg. In moving forward, the cause is normally incorrect placement of the front leg in the initial stance. It is vital that the front knee be bent over the front toe; this way, the body center is already over (or close to being over, depending on femur length) the front foot. This allows the front leg to be in the correct position to begin the drive at the beginning of the movement. As for rear-leg double stepping when moving backward, it is important to think of a contraction movement such as a squeeze of the adductors. The pull backward feels like it comes from the heel.

Shifting

Shifting can be defined as both feet moving in such a way as to shift the body center, only the feet do not change place—the front foot remains the front foot. In addition, in the final position, the feet normally resume their natural-stance position and thus are not wider or narrower than in their initial position. Shifting can take several major forms: yori ashi (sliding), okuri ashi (front foot expanding away from the rear, the rear foot then contracting), and sugi ashi (rear foot stepping up toward the front foot, then the front foot moving forward). These techniques can be performed with elevation, rotation, or vibration as required by a given technique and in a variety of directions or angles.

An additional type of body shifting includes the shifting the body center can undergo when transitioning from one stance to another. For example, by switching from back stance, or kokutsu dachi, to forward stance, or zenkutsu dachi, the body center moves forward as the weight distribution changes from 70/30 (back to front leg, respectively) to 40/60 (back to front leg, respectively).

Dynamics of Yori Ashi

All of the different kinds of shifting are based on exploiting the outward tension of a stance and our natural reflex to catch ourselves when falling.

There are several kinds of yori ashi (sliding techniques). One is okuri ashi, or front foot expanding away from the rear, and rear foot then contracting. Another is sugi ashi, or rear foot stepping up toward the front foot, with the front foot then expanding. These two shifts can be applied to move the body in the front (mae), rear (ushero), or sideways (yoko) directions. For okuri ashi applied in the frontward direction, the initial stance is in outward tension. Next, the leg closest to the direction of movement is lifted and, because of the outward tension of the stance, the leg still connected to the floor pushes the body in the direction of the lifted leg. The lifted leg then drops and connects to the floor, and the rear or pushing leg slides to the length of the initial stance. As both feet connect, outward tension is then applied, allowing the feet to "grab" the floor. Note that this is not a physical push off of the grounded leg, but rather a natural extension of the tension that is already present in the stance. If it does become a push off of the rear leg, the hips will lift during the movement rather than moving parallel to the floor.

In sugi ashi, the rear leg first steps toward the front and acts to drive the front leg outward. This allows a coiling of the rear leg, letting it drive more into the shift, compared to yori or okuri ashi.

Jumping

In tobi, or jumping techniques, both feet leave the ground. These techniques can be very powerful because the full body weight, assisted by gravity, is driving toward the opponent. However, they can be difficult to execute since they are very hard to control, as there is no contact with the ground during flight.

Conclusion

The forces of physics govern all of these translational motions. The formula for momentum is especially important to consider here: $p = mv$. This indicates that in order to create the greatest possible momentum in the technique, the practitioner must create as much velocity as possible, in addition to mass. The easiest way to create velocity is to understand the timing of each point of the step, and know where and when to relax and tense each muscle. Provided this is worked on, there will be no excess tension in the movement, and every muscle contraction will help to move the practitioner to where he or she needs to be and not fight against the movement.

References

Nakayama, M. *Dynamic Karate: Instruction by the Master* Tokyo: Kodansha International, 1966.

Okazaki, T., and M. V. Stricevic. *The Textbook of Modern Karate*. New York: Kodansha International, 1984.

Schmeisser, E. *Advanced Karate-Do*. St. Louis: Focus Publications, 1994.

CHAPTER 16

Rockin' and Rollin': Rotation of the Body to Create Power, Coordination of Movement, and Superior Body Position

Body rotation is an important concept in karate. It means using a rotational movement to create power in a technique. This chapter will describe body rotation in terms of three aspects: (1) joint rotation and creating focus, (2) hip rotation, and (3) body rotation about different axes.

While the kinesiology of rotation will be brought up in other chapters, it is important to remind the reader that angular momentum can be described by the following formula: $L = I\omega$, where

L = angular momentum, I = the moment of inertia (the moment of inertia is resistance to changes in angular velocity, which is directly proportional to mass; for example, it is easier to spin an empty bucket than a full bucket due to the difference in mass), and ω = the angular velocity, which is a product of distance over time. In addition, it can be further defined as $L = r \times mv$, where r = radius of the moment arm, m = mass, and v = velocity. This second formula allows for the conservation of angular momentum. Figure skaters provide a useful analogy here: with their arms out they spin slower, but as they draw their arms in, decreasing their radius, they will start to spin faster. By taking advantage of these physics principles, it is possible to generate vast amounts of force using rotation.

Joint Rotation in Terms of Creating Focus

One important concept, especially with respect to creating finish, or kime, for almost every hand technique, is the full and complete rotation of the radius and ulna of the forearm, and thus the wrist. The wrist can be in one of two positions: either pronated (if the thumb is sticking out like a hitchhiker, it will point toward the body) or supinated (if the thumb is sticking out like a hitchhiker, it will point away from the body). These fully rotated positions cause the muscles in the forearm to flex and, with the clench of the fist, will allow a point of contraction for the entire body.

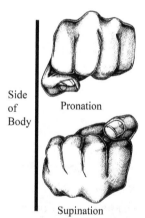

Side of Body

Pronation

Supination

Pronation or supination of the wrist relative to the body.

This concept is involved in almost all karate hand and arm techniques, including oi, gyaku and jun zuki (supination to pronation), gedan barai, age and shuto uke (supination to pronation), and uchi and soto ude uke (pronation to supination). This fast and complete wrist rotation from pronation to supination, or supination to pronation, is key to developing fast and relaxed techniques. The concept is really addressed and concentrated on for the first time in the Tekki series of kata, although in hindsight, it has been practiced from the start of training.

Another important point about wrist rotation is its use in blocking techniques. For example, in the outside cross block, or soto ude uke, it is really the wrist rotation from pronation to supination that provides the finesse of the block, and much of the body movement is involved in getting the arm and body to a reinforced position to be able to make the block. So while the hips rotate to get the body into a half-face hip, or hanmi position, this moves the elbow to the correct one-fist-width distance from the hip. In this dynamic movement, the wrist should still be fully pronated, and the palm side of the wrist will come into contact with the attacking limb. At this point of contact, the body connects and the wrist is quickly rotated to the fully supinated position, effectively changing the contact surface from the "wide, flat" part of the wrist to the "skinny" part of the wrist, shifting the attacking limb. Since this rotation has a very small radius, it is very powerful thanks to the conservation of angular momentum.

Hip Rotation for Generating Power in Techniques

Hip rotation comes about through the half (hanmi) and full (shomen) hip positions. These positions represent the maximum movement allowed by the flexibility of the ball-and-socket joints of the hip and femur. A common misconception is that the hips drive the rotation. Remember that the hip itself has no muscles, so the legs drive the hips, which allows for this motion. As we noted earlier, the movement could be compared to putting two toothpicks into a potato (similar to the femurs, or thigh bones of the legs). If the ends of the toothpicks are manipulated so that one is forward and one is back, the potato will take a hanmi position. If now you push on the rear toothpick, the potato will rotate to the shomen position. Notice that it is not the potato doing the movement but you pushing the toothpicks into position. This is exactly analogous to your legs pushing the hips from the floor into position.

Another important point is that rotation is often thought of as an actual rotation or swinging motion of the hips. While this is technically correct, it is more accurate to think of rotation in terms of expansion and contraction. That is, to get to hanmi, think of the full expansion, push out on the outside edges of the feet, and this will automatically rotate the hips to hanmi. When you go to shomen, think contraction and change the direction of the foot push to out from the toes of the front foot and straight back through the heel of the rear foot. This will contract the hips to shomen automatically. By thinking of the hip rotation as an expansion/contraction rather than a full rotation, the muscles employed change from primarily glutes, quadriceps, and hip flexors to adductors and inductors, which are very fast twitch. (Think of how quickly someone can close their legs when a kick is coming toward their

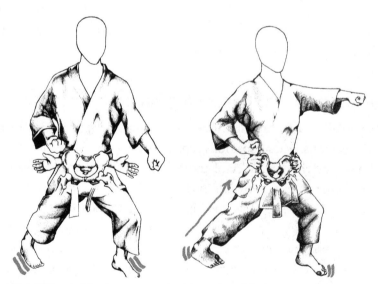

Hip rotation explained as an expansion/contraction of the hips, using the driving leg (shime) to forcibly and quickly rotate the hip forward, similar to closing a door.

groin.) Similar principles govern all stances and reverse half-face hip, or gyaku hanmi positions, but will not be discussed here.

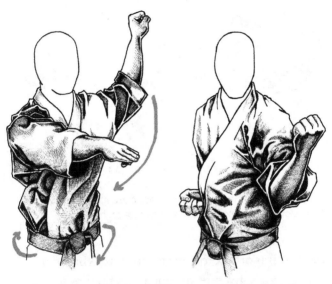

Direct hip rotation using soto ude uke as an example. Note that the elbow moves in the same direction relative to the hip.

While the rotation of the hip uses the same mechanics, two rotations can technically be defined relative to the attacking/ defending limb movement. These can be termed direct rotation and reverse rotation. Direct rotation is when the moving limb is moving in the same direction as the hip. Examples of this include basic soto ude uke, age uke, and kizami zuki. Reverse rotation is when the moving limb is moving in the opposite direction to the hips. Examples include gedan barai, uchi uke, and shuto uke. It is important to point out that this principle and these examples are not mutually exclusive. For example, the last four movements of Heian shodan, the four knife-hand blocks, or shuto uke, involve both direct and reverse rotation. In the first and third blocks (executed from the turns), the rotation of the body mirrors the rotation of the hips, and in classic reverse rotation, the second and forth blocks are simply steps forward. This shows that hip rotation is

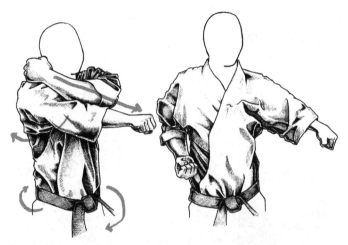

Reverse hip rotation using gedan barai as an example. Note that the elbow moves in the opposite direction relative to the hip.

versatile. It is important to pay attention to what makes the body feel strongest for a given technique in its final position.

Body Rotation in Terms of Axis and Gaining Better Body Position

The final concept covered here is full body rotation in terms of where the axis of rotation is placed. Due to the conservation of angular momentum, it is paramount that nothing should increase the radius of rotation. This means that throughout the rotation the body must remain upright and be moved from the center. If the body bends, the radius will be increased, thus increasing angular momentum. This will make the body much harder to control during the rotation.

The key point here is that one has to be to be aware of the axis of rotation. A common misconception about hip rotation is that there is a single axis of rotation through the backbone. But the axis of rotation can move. For example, when performing reverse punch (gyaku zuki) from a half-face, or hanmi position, the axis should in fact be along the front hip, resulting in a hip action akin to slamming a door. Therefore, as long as the spine remains perpendicular to the floor, the axis can move laterally through the body, depending on need and the drive of the body center.

This axis may be shifted through the body with a clear understanding of the relationship between the rotation, the shift in body center, and the desired outcome of the technique. In the gyaku zuki example above, the rotation of the hip must be in line with the desired outcome. If the rotation occurs through the back hip, the body center will be pulled away from the direction of the technique, thus decreasing the impact to the target. If it is done through the center of the body, rotating using the spine as the central axis, then the body center will not move forward, and there will only be a medium amount of energy delivered to the target since the body mass will not be employed in the technique. However, if the front hip is used as the rotational axis, then the body center will shift in the direction of the target, thus increasing the mass by coupling rotational force with the linear force that can be delivered to the target. While the latter option is superior, it is constrained by the practitioner's flexibility through the back or driving leg. The leg must be able to continue to push off the ground for the duration of the technique and not disconnect from the floor.

This concept of shifting through differential points of the hip— the front, rear, or center of the hip—is technique-specific. The desired outcome of the technique is paramount and should guide where the rotation initiates. For example, in blocking techniques such as soto ude uke, or outside cross block (soto ude uke), from a static position, the outcome of the block can vary dramatically in a dynamic situation. If the rotation happens through the front of the hip, this can have the effect of jamming or driving back the opponent due to the body center moving in, analogous to the collision of two pool balls. If the spine is used as the axis, then the opponent can be deflected at a ninety-degree angle. If the rear hip is used as the rotational axis, then the opponent can be absorbed and pulled off balance in the direction of his attack, as if he were pulled off balance by overstepping.

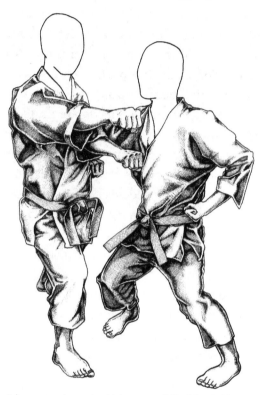

A lunge punch, or oi zuki, is successfully defended by rotating the body and striking with yoko empi uchi.

One of the more extreme examples of changing the rotational axis in karate can be applied to blocking in jiyu kumite, or free sparring. In basic applications, the block is performed by rotating the hips to the hanmi position, with the axis of rotation being the center of the spine. I argue that in situations where the distance between two opponents is not fixed but rather dynamic "floating maai"— where the distance between the two opponents is not fixed—the axis of rotation becomes the lead hand; specifically, the rotating wrist becomes the axis of rotation, and the body moves into position around it. Therefore, in dynamic situations, the karateka needs to be aware of three things: (1) the axis of rotation in respect to their own body, (2) the final location of the body center relative to the opponent (total body position, including angle and distance to the opponent), and (3) the timing of the movement. If all three are taken into account, then it is possible to complete a powerful, smooth transition from defense to attack.

References

Nakayama, M. *Dynamic Karate: Instruction by the Master*. Tokyo: Kodansha International, 1966.

Okazaki, T., and M. V. Stricevic. *The Textbook of Modern Karate*. New York: Kodansha International, 1984.

CHAPTER 17

Breathing: The Key to Coordination

Body expansion and contraction is vital for the coordination of movement in karate. Goran Glucina, seventh dan SKIF, commented that "karate is the most natural thing for your body; it as simple as breathing." This comment is extremely insightful. Body expansion and contraction refers to the movement from one position to another with good timing. The timing is controlled through breath. In this chapter, we will break down some of the components of breathing, body connection, and expansion and contraction. Initially, we will discuss relaxation and the contraction and expansion of movement, then we will move to the concept of timing. From there we will talk about the ways in which timing can be controlled through breath. Finally, we will see how good control of expansion and contraction of movements as controlled by breath connects to concepts such as kiai and kime.

Throughout this chapter, we will be using some terms that are important to put into context here. Expansion refers to having a limb in some fully extended position, while contraction refers to the initial movement of that limb or body part, such as the hips, from that position (like letting go of a rubber band). Body expansion and body contraction refer to the whole-body feel of a movement. For example, in lower block, or gedan barai, the final position of the movement is in full-body expansion while the load for the block is in full-body contraction. But the concept can get a little more complicated. When one moves from the fully expanded (and body-expanded) movement of gedan barai (left figure below), the arm movement initially contracts to bring the elbows together for the preparatory position (middle figure). When in the preparatory position, the body is contracted, but other muscles in the load position are now expanded (lengthened) and can be used in our rubber band analogy to initiate the following technique (right figure). Another term referred to here is tensing. This is often at the full, final body-expanded or body-contracted positions, but at more advanced levels can be separated from them.

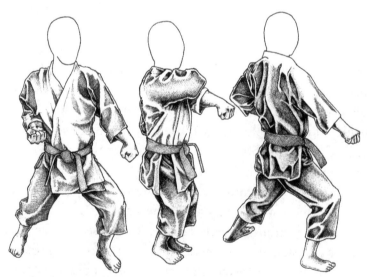

Stepping forward from the expanded zenkutsu gedan barai (forward stance lower sweep) with the left leg forward, to the expanded zenkutsu gedan barai with the right leg forward. The middle figure is the contracted preparatory position.

Oftentimes this contraction is called kime, but as we will see, it encapsulates a much larger concept and will be discussed separately below.

Relaxation and the Contraction and Expansion of Movement

The flow from one movement to another can be likened to a rubber band. The flow from one movement to another is from full-body expansion in one direction to full-body expansion in another direction. A simple example of this is stepping from gedan barai to gedan barai (see illustration in the last section). Through the course of the movement, the practitioner steps from a full-body-expanded position to a body contraction through the center, which stretches muscles in the opposite direction and then moves to another fully expanded position. In order to achieve this movement smoothly, karateka can make use of the elasticity of their tendons. By dynamically stepping into the first gedan barai at full expansion, the tendons are stretched 15 percent of their length as the muscle contracts. As they spring back to their normal length, the practitioner can use that tendon contraction to initiate the next step while contracting the hips and arms to a fully compressed state and then allowing the natural tendon contraction to initiate the movement in the opposite direction. This type of movement is exactly analogous to a counter jump (the little jump people often use to initiate a large dynamic movement).

A stretched rubber band offers a good analogy. You use the energy gained from the stretch to initiate the next movement, which again stretches the rubber band in another direction, which in turn is used to initiate the next stretch, and so on.

This springy, tensile movement allows both the smooth transition from one technique to another and the quick timing between movements. For example, if you execute gedan barai hard and strong in zenkutsu dachi while allowing the limbs to be at full expansion and then you immediately relax, your body will move slightly in the direction of the next technique. This allows your hips to naturally start to rotate your body for the next contraction as it accelerates to gyaku zuki. In order for this to happen, a few conditions have to be in place. First, the movement must be relaxed throughout, with tensing only when required, which, when the distance between the two opponents is not fixed, is at the ends of the movements, or at the point where contact would be made with an opponent. Second, the tensing winds the muscles into a full-body expansion or contraction movement. Third, all of this movement needs to be timed correctly.

Timing

Timing refers to the general coordination of movements as a single unit. In karate this is often described as the feet and hands moving together. However, this can be better defined as the body center and hips moving together with one or more limbs. Coordinating movement through the body center is vital to correct body expansion and contraction. If the limbs are moving in an uncoordinated fashion relative to one another or the body center, the movement as a whole will be ineffective. To do this, it is important to think through the body center first and foremost, best described by Steve Ubl (eighth dan, WTKO) as "put your eyes and look through your center point."

In a perfect world, the feet, arms, and hips all stop moving at the same time. This applies not only to the conclusion of the movement, but should be considered throughout the movement. For example, in stepping forward from zenkutsu dachi with gedan barai to zenkutsu dachi again with gedan barai, the entire movement needs the hands, feet, and body center to move in turn, starting from the full-body-expanded position, to the full-body-contracted position (the preparatory position), to the full-body-expanded position, together. In particular, the full-body contraction (preparatory position) has both arms wrapped around the front of the neck, and the feet are together and squeezed all at the same instant before the movement changes to the expansion phase.

A way to remember this is to imagine that the elbow of the rear hand and the knee of the rear leg are connected by a piece of string. The elbow and knee move as a single unit throughout the movement. Unfortunately, this type of coordinated movement is very difficult to put into practice, especially when coordinating opposite arms and feet. Therefore, breath is often used.

Breath

Breath in karate is inextricably linked to the expansion and contraction of karate movement, as well as to the coordination of these movements. In addition, it allows connection and tensing of the muscles in a coordinated fashion. At a very basic level, inhalation is often used to relax, and is joined with body contraction. Exhalation, on the other hand, is joined with body expansion, and is often used to help with the final tensing of muscles and to engage intra-abdominal pressure (IAP) (see chapter 14).

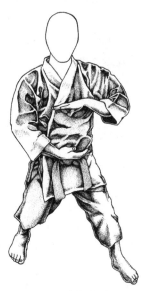

Contraction of the body center through breath, resulting in IAP.

In the example of stepping forward from zenkutsu dachi with gedan barai to zenkutsu dachi with gedan barai, the inhalation is timed to the movement from full-body expansion to full-body contraction (to the preparatory position), then the exhalation is coordinated with the full-body contraction to the full-body expansion (preparatory position to execution).

An additional point to make here is that the use of IAP is not necessarily associated with an outward breath. Recall that IAP is created by contracting the abdominals and the rectus (inward) and flexing the diaphragm. Remember also that with an outward breath the diaphragm flexes down and creates pressure on the viscera. It is also possible to create the same downward pressure by filling the lungs with air. Therefore, IAP can be achieved on either inward or outward breaths.

It is also important to note that IAP does not require a full exhalation. In the example of gedan braai to gyaku zuki, IAP can be employed twice on the same out-breath. As the block is executed, the breath is exhaled and stopped using IAP as the technique makes contact with the opponent. The diaphragm is immediately relaxed, and the exhalation is continued as the punch is executed, where again IAP is used as the punch makes contact. This principle can be used to allow for multiple techniques in a single out-breath and can be used to string techniques together.

Finally, if multiple techniques are used in a single exhalation, one can make use of the diaphragm and natural expansion and contraction of the chest that occurs during IAP to extend the breath. As the technique is executed and IAP is employed, the chest will naturally contract. As the diaphragm is relaxed immediately after the technique is executed, the chest expands a little, creating a slight vacuum that allows a small amount of air to enter the lungs before the exhalation continues. This type of breathing is called pulse breathing, and it can greatly increase the number of techniques that can be executed on the single breath.

The above principles can then be extrapolated: while the breath is moving, the body is in movement, but when the breath stops (allowing for IAP), the muscles of the limbs need to be contracted, either in full-body expansion or in full-body contraction (which normally coincides with contact with the opponent). An important point is that while every technique has some form of hip movement to add power to the technique, each technique also has a breath component that coordinates the movement overall. The two are joined together.

Kiai and Kime

The concepts of kiai (visceral shout) and kime (decision or focus) are linked to these concepts. In addition, the two are linked to one another. The kiai is a product of the kime, and the kime is aided by the kiai.

Kime is the complete focus of an execution of a technique from beginning to end, resulting in the perfect finish. It encapsulates not just the end point of the technique, but the entire path used to execute the technique. It also incorporates the three major areas of body, mind, and spirit.

In terms of the body, kime is about achieving the correct outward form of the technique, the correct shape and body alignment. The body should also have the correct internal form, correct timing, correct application of IAP, and correct breathing. This body aspect includes the concept of timed body expansion and body contraction. The mind aspect can be thought of as focusing both on what is happening externally to the body and on what is happening internally. The external mental aspect involves control of the mind to place the attacking limb at the right place at the right time and to calculate how to do it against a moving target. It is the mechanical ability to focus and coordinate a limb on a single point in space. Internally, the mind is coordinating everything: the neuromuscular pathways to move the limbs, the breath, and coordination. The spirit aspect is about actually wanting to hit the target and having the emotional focus and will to drive into the target. All of this must be coordinated in some fashion, and breath plays that role. By coordinating the breath with the movement, we have a way to move from the body center using IAP and harmonize our techniques with mind and spirit.

When all of this comes together with breath, a sound is produced: the kiai. Kiai is of two words: ki meaning energy and ai meaning bringing together. Therefore, a kiai is the noise produced when you have complete coordination, both internally and externally, of the body, mind, and spirit, using breath and body center to focus on a single point in space during the impact of a technique.

Conclusion

Based on this chapter, it is obvious how important the concepts of expansion and contraction are in karate, and, more importantly, how they are inextricably linked to timing, breath, and IAP. Timing, breath, and IAP provide much of the link between how we need both mass (tensing, or kime) and acceleration (complete relaxation) coupled together to produce force in techniques. More importantly, breath can clearly be used as the central controlling factor to coordinate these factors together in our techniques. Therefore, karate really is the most natural thing for your body—as simple as breathing.

References

Nakayama, M. *Dynamic Karate: Instruction by the Master.* Tokyo: Kodansha International, 1966.

Norris, C. M. "Abdominal Muscle Training in Sport," *Br J Sp Med* **27** (1993): 19–27.

Okazaki, T., and M. V. Stricevic. *The Textbook of Modern Karate.* New York: Kodansha International, 1984.

Schmeisser, E. *Advanced Karate-Do.* St. Louis: Focus Publications, 1994.

CHAPTER 18

How Do I Hit Things and Not Fall Over? Keage, Kekomi, and Ate

Reaction force is a vital component of karate techniques. This chapter will discuss the concept in two ways. The first is how reaction force can be used to hit the target to achieve different results. The second is the internal reaction force often used to balance or reinforce the body.

How Do I Hit Things?

According to physics, when you push against a wall or hit a target (action force), the target will push back into you with an equal amount of force until either the force applied stops or either side gives way. In addition, it can take time to transfer that action force, and for the object getting force applied to it to transfer that force back into the force applier (reaction force). In karate, we try to apply the maximum amount of force to the target as quickly as possible. However, the way we apply action force and deal with the reaction force can vary depending on technique. In short, in Shotokan karate we have three major ways we can hit things (note that this does not count deflection, used to block). They are keage, or snap; kekomi, or thrust; and ate or smash.

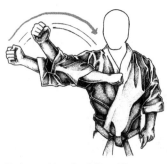

Uraken uchi, or backfist strike, as an example of keage. Note the strong emphasis on the retraction of the technique.

Keage

Keage, or snap, is typified by side snap kick, or yoko geri keage, and backfist strike, or uraken uchi. In these techniques, the limb penetrates the target, pushing through the soft tissue layers, then immediately retracts before the opposing body applies reaction force to the attacking limb. This is achieved through a snapping motion, where the retraction is the highest priority, similar to snapping a towel. A common ratio is 30 percent effort driving the technique outward and 70 percent effort snapping the technique back. This type of attack causes the reaction force as well as the attacking force to be dissipated into the opponent, since the practitioner absorbs little or no reaction force. Generally, the opponent will not be forced back by the technique, but will rather vibrate in place as they absorb the shock or will collapse straight downward.

This type of action may be seen if you are sitting in the bathtub and have your hand placed on the surface of the water. Quickly drop your hand downward, and there will be a momentary hole in the water where your hand has pushed through. This hole is analogous to the effect of the snap and retraction of the attacking limb on soft tissue. Note how the water slaps together very violently as it refills the hole left behind by your hand.

Due to there being little or no reaction force applied to the attacker, there is little or no need to reinforce the technique through one's body. While intra-abdominal pressure still connects the limb to the floor, there is no need for strong reinforcement through the body.

Quite often the concept of keage can be mistaken as referring only to striking techniques: techniques that hit the target at an angle perpendicular to the long bone of the striking limb. However, thrusting techniques can also be keage-like. As long as the concept of fast retraction is employed, the same result will come about.

Kekomi

Kekomi, or thrust, can be seen in the examples of side thrust kick (yoko geri kekomi) and lunge punch (oi zuki). In these techniques, the attacking limb is driven and locked into place approximately one fist length into the target for a few microseconds longer than keage. The attacker absorbs the reaction force and has a clear body alignment with the floor. For example, in the final position of oi zuki finishing in forward stance, or zenkutsu dachi, there is a clear path from the fist, along the straight arm, to the connected shoulder and back, to the connected hip and rear buttock, to the extended straight leg, and finally to the heel connected to the floor. This body position is reinforced and therefore hopefully stronger than the reaction force of the opponent, causing all force to be transferred to the opponent, and the opposing reaction force from the opponent to go through the attacker's body (if in correct alignment), hit the rooted heel on the floor, and bounce back through the attacker's body into the opponent. If there is correct body alignment, the attacker should feel nothing as the force is transferred; however, if there is poor body alignment, the attacker

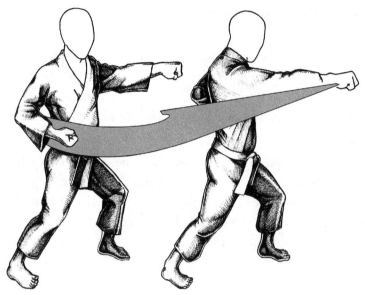

Gyaku zuki as an example of kekomi. Note how the body needs to reinforce the technique through the straight driving rear leg.

will feel the break at the responsible joint, and energy that could otherwise go into the attacker will be dissipated at that joint. Therefore, it is crucial to have good reinforcement of the attacking technique and good body alignment.

Penetration and the speed of the technique are important in kekomi. The attacking limb must be moving at full speed when it penetrates the target. This obeys the law of $F = ma$ (force = mass × acceleration), which implies that in order to apply the maximum amount of force to an object, the force-applying object must be accelerating as much as possible, and then the amount of mass behind it must be maximized as well. This means keeping the technique as relaxed as possible, and only when the limb has penetrated the target should the muscles be locked up for a very brief period of time. This is the concept of kime, or "perfect finish." Often, students will not be relaxed, resulting in a slowing of the technique and reduction of the force applied to the target.

A common mistake is that people often leave the technique extended for too long in kekomi. So how long should the technique be extended into the target? The length of time the leg should be extended in keage versus in kekomi techniques has been best defined by Matthew Pain, PhD, a professor in the School of Sport, Exercise and Health Sciences at Loughborough University and fifth dan, Fudochi Karate, UK. He comments, using yoko geri as an example, that in keage the foot should snap out and back so that your eye is unable to focus on your toenails. For kekomi, your eye is able to focus on them ever so briefly before the leg is snapped back. Considering that the eye can typically focus in 350 milliseconds, the leg is not extended in kekomi for long.

Ate

Ate, or smashing techniques, are literally designed to go through the opponent. Some examples are morote uke (applied as a strike),

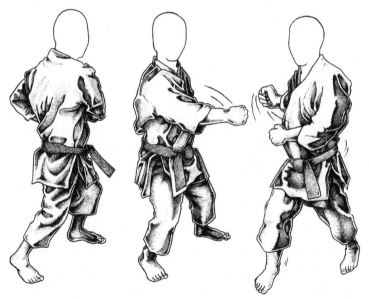

Using the hips to swing the arm in an uraken uchi, or backfist strike, through the target as an example of ate.

mae empi uchi, and mawashi empi uchi. In these types of techniques, the striking limb is locked in place, and the rest of the body continues to drive completely through the target. This could be likened to swinging a baseball bat. These types of techniques rely on creating a large amount of momentum moving the body weight through a weak vector or a target (e.g., on a thirty-degree angle in a front stance). Once again, it is hoped that the generated body momentum will overcome the reaction force that can be applied back into the attacker.

Using Breath to Control Keage, Kekomi, and Ate

Instructors notice that lower-ranked students tend to lock up at the end of their technique. In the previous chapter we discussed breath in relation to the perfect finish, or kime. Here we discuss it in connection to the actual contact with the opponent.

The sequence of the techniques like keage, kekomi, and ate from execution to target impact will generally not vary. What will vary is what one does immediately afterward, and this depends on what effect the attacker wishes to achieve. General rules, such as the body center moving toward the target, correct alignment of the body, reinforcement of the body if needed, and coordination of breath to form intra-abdominal pressure (IAP) and kime, must all be upheld. However, immediately following the impact phase of the technique there is variation. As discussed above, a keage technique immediately and sharply retracts from the target, kekomi very briefly locks in place, and ate continues to drive through the target. The question, however, is how this is coordinated.

The answer is through breathing. To allow smooth flow from one technique to another, the previous technique needs to be immediately relaxed. This is achieved by immediately inhaling after IAP. As one creates IAP, the abdominals and diaphragm are compressed downward, resulting in a cessation of breathing. The quickest way to release this contraction is to immediately breathe in. Therefore, the ability to execute and transition among keage, kekomi, and ate is in how this in-breath is performed.

In short, the in-breath must mirror the technique being executed. Once kime is achieved and the attack has penetrated the target, the force and speed for the next inhalation must mirror the type of hit. A short, very sharp inhalation coupled with the correct body motion, in this case a sharp retraction, results in keage. A slightly longer in-breath results in kekomi, while no stop in the out-breath (you literally breathe through the opponent), results in ate. Thus, the in-breath controls the tempo and nature of the technique.

Internal Reaction Force

Internal reaction force refers to the internal feeling of the technique as it is executed. We have already described correct alignment of the body, so here the focus will be on hikite, or the forceful retraction of the opposing limb. As we have stated throughout this chapter, Newton's third law indicates that for every forward motion there must be an equal and opposite reactive motion. When moving the body in techniques such as choku zuki, it can be instructive to use the opposite limb to "balance out" the technique. This concept is vital for focusing the body into a single unit at the point of impact. In addition, by focusing on the retraction, the attacking limb will become more relaxed, allowing for greater speed of the attacking limb. Eventually (after many years), the

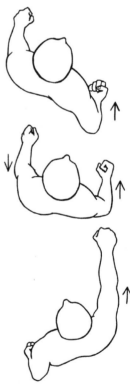

Use of hikite in balancing out a punching technique.

physical hikite can be removed from the technique (within reason), as long as the feeling is still present. Finally, hikite is involved in many applied variations in techniques. This can include grabbing and pulling motions.

Conclusion

Reaction force is very important in karate, primarily in terms of how we interact with our opponent. In short, we endeavor to manipulate our opponent's reaction force with methods including keage, kekomi, and ate. Finally, we also use our own reaction force to ensure correct direction of force into a target.

References

Mitchell, D. *Official Karate*. London: Stanley Paul, 1986.

Nakayama, M. *Best Karate*. Tokyo: Kodansha International, 1977.

Nakayama, M. *Dynamic Karate: Instruction by the Master*. Tokyo: Kodansha International, 1966.

Okazaki, T., and M. V. Stricevic. *The Textbook of Modern Karate*. New York: Kodansha International, 1984.

Schmeisser, E. *Advanced Karate-Do*. St. Louis: Focus Publications, 1994.

CHAPTER 19

Is There Equipment That Can Help Me?

Much of modern karate training can be done simply by refining one's technique through careful internal reflection. The only thing required is a karate uniform, or do-gi. However, there can be great benefit to using equipment in training. The use of equipment can be vital for developing a method of direct feedback regarding the execution and delivery of power into a target. To this end, equipment can be used for two primary purposes: (1) understanding the internal feeling of the body as a technique impacts an object, and (2) developing focus and power delivery through correct alignment to a target outside the body.

While what we discuss here is not an exhaustive list, I intend to focus on several vital methodologies and apparatus that are in common use in most modern dojo (1–9). In addition, the benefits of training equipment for conditioning the body are beyond the scope of this chapter and are discussed elsewhere in the literature.

Apparatus to Help Develop Internal Feedback

One of the key aspects of all karate training is to develop internal connection as well as correct body alignment of arms and legs. This is sometimes known as intra-abdominal pressure (IAP), which we have discussed at length. To review, IAP occurs when the muscles of the lower abdomen, stomach, and back flex to create the walls of a box. Next, the karate practitioner breathes in such a way as to flex the diaphragm down to put pressure on the internal viscera, which pushes out on the walls of the box to make it solid. It is through this solid box that karate practitioners can connect their arms to the floor to generate power. Unfortunately, without feedback in some way—just training by punching the air, for example— the practitioner may be unable to develop this kind of body feeling.

Weights and Weight Training

One way to develop this type of feeling is to use light weights (one to five pounds max) or sai,[8] in the hands, on the ankles, or on the trunk, increasing the weight over time. Or a five- to fifteen-pound weight vest could be employed, using slow-motion techniques. This extra weight at the end of a lever causes the internal muscles to flex, and if practitioners pay attention to their body, they can get a feel for the contractions required by the various movements for karate. This will also allow the practitioner to become aware of the deep muscle contractions vital to proper technique. It is paramount that the practitioner use light weights, as anything too heavy will cause the incorrect muscles to be used; the weights should just serve as an amplifier for normal unweighted movement.

---

8. A sai is a traditional weapon used in Okinawan martial arts. It is traditionally a three-pronged metal truncheon on which all three prongs extend from the handle and point forward. The center prong is normally longer than the flanking two.

Partner

Another incredibly useful piece of training equipment is the partner. A partner can provide immediate feedback on techniques as they are executed. One partner-based technique widely used in other types of karate (Goju-ryu and Uechi-ryu) is shime. This is often employed during the practice of Sanchin kata, where trainees are slapped and pushed as they contract throughout the movement. This provides direct feedback on stability as well as on core and limb connection to that core. In Shotokan, we have only a single kata that can compare to the isometric heavy feeling of Sanchin. That is the kata Hangetsu. However, if we modify this type of training to achieve quick execution and release, characteristic of many Shotokan movements, we can derive benefits.

To do this, the same slapping motions (to the abdomen, back muscles, arms) can be used at the point of connection to see if the karateka is in fact using the correct muscles at the correct time.

Obi

One invaluable tool for developing internal feedback is the belt, or obi. It is important to wear the obi reasonably tight so that the compression of the abdomen can be felt against the ring of the obi. In normal technique we want the abdomen to be at 30 percent pressure against the obi; however, during the impact phase you want 100 percent pressure for that instant.

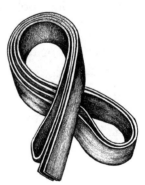

The karate obi. A very useful tool in developing karate technique.

Impact Training

Impact training is important for understanding internal connection. For this, two major pad types are used: flexible light pads, such as clappers and hand-held focus mitts, and solid hard pads,

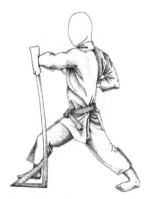

Use of the makiwara in developing karate technique.

such as body shields, heavy bags, partners with phone books in their gi, and punching posts, or makiwara. The latter is important for both internal and external connection and will be addressed in the next section as well as here.

As one strikes a solid target, the target provides force directly back into the body, proportional to the force applied to the target. The force applied back can provide invaluable feedback regarding body connection, alignment, the use of intra-abdominal pressure, and the timing of all these related to the striking of the target. In order to get the maximum amount of feedback, it is important to hit a solid target that provides some flex, so as not to damage the body part striking it. Common apparatus include traditional makiwara, hung punching bags, and partners holding body shields and focus mitts. If the club does not have access to any of these items, a phone book placed inside the front of the karate gi may be used.

When hitting the target, it is important that the practitioner feel the impact traverse directly through the practitioner's body to the heel in contact with the floor. If impact or give is felt in any joint (wrist, elbow, shoulder, lower back, knee, or ankle), it is an immediate indication that the practitioner does not have correct body alignment.

Apparatus to Help Develop External Feedback

In addition to understanding how it feels to hit a target, it is also important to understand how to hit the target. This includes being able to do the calculus for correct targeting, technique, timing, and distance to the target.

Obi

One very useful piece of apparatus is the obi. The obi can be folded lengthwise in half, then in half again. One partner can then hold it in one hand approximately one foot down from the loop end. The folded obi then can represent a one- to two-inch midline from the top of the head to the bottom of the torso. The other partner can then kick, strike, and punch one to two inches into the obi, with good kime.

Impact Apparatus

The use of pads, bags, and punching posts, or makiwara, are also useful for developing external feedback. It is important to have a percussive shock when striking the target, as this represents sharp kime. Quite often when striking targets, it can be easy to get sucked into the idea that a hard push is the same as a strike. Unfortunately, while feeling strong, a push can use antagonistic muscles that slow the technique and thus reduce the impact power.

If practitioners find themselves doing this, they need to adjust their distance back away from the target so that they just strike the surface of the pad. Once this is achieved, the practitioner may then gradually strike deeper into the pad, maintaining that feeling up to the distance equivalent to the length of their fist, approximately two to three inches. If at any point the technique becomes a push rather than a shock, the process needs to be repeated.

An impact pad is also useful to distinguish keage techniques from kekomi techniques. When a pad or individual is hit with a keage technique, they should vibrate and stop dead where they are, while a kekomi technique should knock the pad or individual back on the same vector the technique is employed along.

Conclusion

While the use of air training is vital for identifying the correct course of movement, it is important to gain feedback from external sources. This helps the practitioner discern internal and external feelings within techniques. The training equipment I have discussed here is widely available and can be very beneficial to one's training.

Notes

1. D. L. Bartelink, "The Role of Abdominal Pressure in Relieving the Pressure on the Lumbar Intervertebral Discs," *J Bone Joint Surg* **39-B** (1957): 718–725.
2. G. Funakoshi, *Karate Do Kyohan: Master Text for the Way of the Empty Hand* (San Diego: Neptune Publications, 2005).
3. H. Kanazawa, *S.K.I. Kumite Kyohan* (Tokyo: SKI, 1987).
4. M. Nakayama, *Dynamic Karate: Instruction by the Master* (Tokyo: Kodansha International, 1966), 308.
5. T. Okazaki and M. V. Stricevic, *The Textbook of Modern Karate* (New York: Kodansha International, 1984).
6. H. Nishiyama and R. C. Brown, *Karate: The Art of "Empty-Hand" Fighting* (Boston: Tuttle Publishing, 1960).
7. E. Schmeisser, *Advanced Karate-Do* (St. Louis: Focus Publications, 1994).
8. P. Urban, *The Karate Dojo: Traditions and Tales of a Martial Art* (Rutland, VT: Tuttle Publishing, 1967), 145.
9. G. Yamaguchi, *Goju Ryu Karate Do Kyohan* (Hamilton, ON: Masters Publication, 1999).

CHAPTER 20

Conclusion

This book is dedicated to the correct execution of karate movements. Initial discussion concerned external techniques of karate. This included weapons of the body, postures, and techniques such as thrusts, strikes, kicks, blocks, and unbalancing an opponent. Next, fundamental biology and biomechanics were addressed and applied to karate. Finally, the subtler internal movements were examined. In particular, these movements were applied to the execution of karate and included hip motion, center connection, breathing, how targets are hit, and the physical apparatus that can help us develop better karate.

One of the major concepts explored throughout this book is the interrelationship of intra-abdominal pressure, breathing, timing, hip vibration, and kime. Traditionally, hip vibration was classified, along with body shifting and hip rotation, as one of the ways to generate power through the movement of the hips. Given our examination of this concept, I assert that "hip vibration" is a misleading term, and what it describes arguably does not really exist. Therefore, I suggest that we replace "hip vibration" with the term "core compression," which much more adequately encapsulates the body feeling. Core compression is achieved via the application of breath and IAP, and can result in a powerful motion of the hips as the torso compresses. This connects the arms and legs to the torso for the instant one is in physical contact with an opponent. In addition, core compression is used in conjunction with all other hip motions, including all aspects of shifting and rotation. And while core compression is initiated with the movement, it provides the final connection, or kime, of the technique.

Examples have been provided throughout this book to illustrate various concepts that are often not well described elsewhere. Where possible, I have provided analogies or training methods that help you to understand each concept. The next step is for you to take these ideas and integrate them into your own training in order to make progress. If you pay attention to both gross and micro-level body movement and meticulously correct each part according to

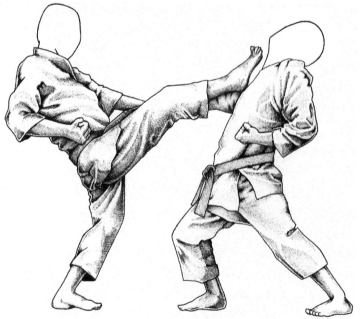

Jodan mae geri, or upper-level front kick.

the principles discussed in this book, your body will develop the correct neuromuscular pathways. Slowly, over time, your karate will improve. Kanazawa Hirokazu (tenth dan SKIF) has often been identified as the source of the quote, "Practice does not make perfect; only perfect practice makes perfect."

Central to this entire book has been the four major principles that allow one to prefect his or her karate movement. These principles—good posture, good alignment, good body mechanics, and good practical functionality—are all prerequisites for correct karate movement and must be continuously developed through training. It is my hope that this book will help you think about these principles and how to integrate them into your training to aid the development of your karate technique.

Make your karate practice perfect.

INDEX

Note that tsuki is used by itself, while zuki is used when the word is joined to a
name (i.e., tsuki = thrusting techniques; oi-zuki = stepping punch).

Note that keri is used by itself, while geri is used when the word is joined to a name
(i.e., keri = kicking techniques; mae-geri = front kick).

ABOUT THE AUTHOR

J. D. SWANSON, PhD, is an associate professor in the Department of Biology and Biomedical Sciences at Salve Regina University in Newport, Rhode Island. He currently has a successful federally funded research program working on novel treatments for stomach cancer. In addition, he teaches classes in anatomy and physiology, genetics, cell biology, kinesiology, and developmental biology. He recently wrote and implemented a new course at Salve Regina that uses 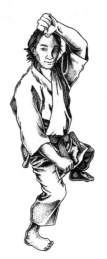 karate as a conduit for teaching fundamental freshman pedagogical skills (writing, researching, and reading). This class spends equal time on the dojo floor and in the classroom, and it covers basic karate as well as its history, biomechanics, and philosophy.

Dr. Swanson began his karate training in 1980 in his hometown in New Zealand. There he passed dan examinations in the SKIF (Kanazawa) faction of Shotokan karate, as well as his dan examinations in taekwondo (ITF). Upon moving to the United States in 1998, he founded the Pennsylvania State University Shotokan Karate club, which eventually became one of the largest collegiate clubs in the United States. He relocated to Arkansas for a five-year period, during which he was asked to serve as the ISKF Southern Region Director with Mr. Leon Sill for the International Shotokan Karate Federation (ISKF) after the ISKF/JKA political split in 2007. He moved to New England in 2011.

He has trained continuously from 1980 to the present, and is currently ranked godan in the International Shotokan Karate Federation (tested by Okazaki Teruyuki and Yaguchi Yutaka). He is a graduate of the ISKF Kenshusei course, making him an official instructor, examiner, and judge (details can be found at http://www.iskf.com /information.html). He is the director of the North American Collegiate

Karate Association. He also serves as the instructor for both the Brown University and Salve Regina Shotokan Karate clubs in Rhode Island.

Dr. Swanson has trained all over the world and for significant periods of time with many senior karate instructors, including Okazaki Teruyuki, Yaguchi Yutaka, Kanazawa Hirokazu, Mikami Takayuki, James Field, Robin Rielly, Najib Amin, Cathy Cline, Leon Sill, Okazaki Hiroyoshi, Gary Swain, Steve Ubl, and Goran Glucina. He has also attended seminars headed by some of the best martial arts instructors in the world. In addition to predominantly training in Shotokan and taekwondo dojo, he has also trained periodically with Isshin-ryu, Uechi-ryu, Goju-ryu, judo, aikido, shinkendo, jujitsu, and many other dojo over his karate career.

ABOUT THE ILLUSTRATOR

SAM NIGRO is a medical illustrator who graduated from Salve Regina University with a bachelor's degree in visual arts and a minor in biology. She spent her college career utilizing her education to make visuals of human anatomy and genetic processes. During her junior year, she collaborated with Dr. J. D. Swanson to help her biological artwork achieve accuracy. Her last year was spent juggling a senior thesis of artwork depicting cancer development along with illustrating this book. Today she works as a medical concierge in the emergency department and as a freelance illustrator. She plans to apply to a graduate program in medical illustration within the next two years.

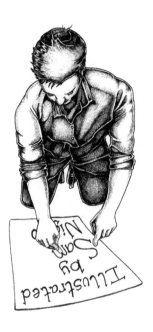

BOOKS FROM YMAA

DVDS FROM YMAA

more products available from . . .

YMAA Publication Center, Inc. 楊氏東方文化出版中心

1-800-669-8892 • info@ymaa.com • www.ymaa.com